DATE DUE			
OCT 23 '92			
DEC 4 '82			
JUL 15 '94			
FEB 17 '95			
OCT 25 1996			
NOV 8 96			
FEB 28 '97			
ILL william			
OCT 03 97			

JUVENILE HOMICIDE

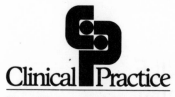

Clinical Practice

The Clinical Practice Series
Number 7

Judith H. Gold, M.D., F.R.C.P.(C)
Series Editor

JUVENILE HOMICIDE

Edited by

ELISSA P. BENEDEK, M.D.
Clinical Professor of Psychiatry, University of Michigan; and Director of Training and Evaluation, Center for Forensic Psychiatry, Ann Arbor, Michigan

DEWEY G. CORNELL, Ph.D.
Assistant Professor, Institute of Clinical Psychology, Curry School of Education, University of Virginia, Charlottesville, Virginia

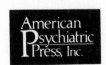

1400 K Street, N.W.
Washington, DC 20005

Copyright © 1989 American Psychiatric Press, Inc.
ALL RIGHTS RESERVED
Manufactured in the United States of America

92 91 90 89 4 3 2 1

The paper used in this publication meets the minimum requirements of the American National Standard for Information Sciences—Permanence of Paper for Printed Library Materials ANSI Z39.48-1984.   ∞

Library of Congress Cataloging-in-Publication Data

Juvenile homicide / edited by Elissa P. Benedek, Dewey G. Cornell.
    p.   cm.—(The Clinical practice series; no. 7)
  Includes bibliographies.
  ISBN 0-88048-145-5 (alk. paper)
  1. Juvenile homicide—Psychological aspects.   2. Forensic psychiatry.   3. Adolescent psychotherapy.   4. Juvenile homicide—United States.   I. Benedek, Elissa P.   II. Cornell, Dewey G.   III. Series: Clinical practice series (Washington, D.C.); no. 7.
  [DNLM: 1. Child Psychiatry.   2. Criminal Psychology.
3. Homicide.   4. Juvenile Delinquency. HV 9067.H6 J97]
RJ506.H65J88 1989
614′.1—dc19
DNLM/DLC
for Library of Congress   88-7682
                                                             CIP

Contents

Contributors

David M. Benedek
Research Assistant, Center for Forensic Psychology, Ann Arbor, Michigan

Elissa P. Benedek, M.D.
Clinical Professor of Psychiatry, University of Michigan; and Director of Training and Evaluation, Center for Forensic Psychiatry, Ann Arbor, Michigan

Richard J. Bonnie, L.L.B.
Professor of Law and Director, Institute of Law, Psychiatry, and Public Policy, University of Virginia, Charlottesville, Virginia

Dewey G. Cornell, Ph.D.
Assistant Professor, Institute of Clinical Psychology, Curry School of Education, University of Virginia, Charlottesville, Virginia

Spencer Eth, M.D.
Assistant Professor of Psychiatry, UCLA School of Medicine; Clinical Associate Professor of Psychiatry, University of Southern California School of Medicine; and Associate Chief of Psychiatry for Ambulatory Care, Veterans Administration Medical Center, Los Angeles, California

W. Lawrence Fitch, J.D.
Director, Forensic Evaluation, Training, and Research Center; Director of Forensic Psychiatry Clinic; and Assistant

Professor of Law, Institute of Law, Psychiatry, and Public Policy, University of Virginia, Charlottesville, Virginia

Gregory B. Leong, M.D.
Psychiatric Consultant, Los Angeles County Superior Court; Assistant Professor of Psychiatry in Residence, School of Medicine, University of California, Los Angeles; and Staff Psychiatrist, West Los Angeles Veterans Administration Medical Center, Los Angeles, California

Donald J. Scherl, M.D.
President and Professor of Psychiatry, State University of New York Health Sciences Center at Brooklyn, Brooklyn, New York

Lois Staresina, A.M.L.S.
Librarian and Research Assistant, Center for Forensic Psychology, Ann Arbor, Michigan

Introduction
to the Clinical Practice Series

Over the years of its existence the series of monographs entitled *Clinical Insights* gradually became focused on providing current, factual, and theoretical material of interest to the clinician working outside of a hospital setting. To reflect this orientation, the name of the Series has been changed to *Clinical Practice*.

The Clinical Practice Series will provide readers with books that give the mental health clinician a practical clinical approach to a variety of psychiatric problems. These books will provide up-to-date literature reviews and emphasize the most recent treatment methods. Thus, the publications in the Series will interest clinicians working both in psychiatry and in the other mental health professions.

Each year a number of books will be published dealing with all aspects of clinical practice. In addition, from time to time when appropriate, the publications may be revised and updated. Thus, the Series will provide quick access to relevant and important areas of psychiatric practice. Some books in the Series will be authored by a person considered to be an expert in that particular area; others will be edited by such an expert who will also draw together other knowledgeable authors to produce a comprehensive overview of that topic.

Some of the books in the Clinical Practice Series will have their foundation in presentations at an Annual Meeting of the American Psychiatric Association. All will contain the most recently available information on the subjects discussed. Theoretical and scientific data will be applied to clinical situations, and case illustrations will be utilized in order to make the material even more relevant for the practitioner. Thus, the Clinical Practice Series should provide educational reading in a compact format especially written for the mental health clinician–psychiatrist.

This monograph, edited by Drs. Benedek and Cornell, discusses the difficult topic of juvenile homicide. The various authors, through discussion of research findings, theory, and actual case examples, illustrate the situations encountered by clinicians as they attempt to successfully diagnose, assess, and advise the court when juveniles are brought before it. Different aspects of all of these are highlighted, and the difficulties involved at every stage are outlined in detail. The clinician who deals with such cases in practice will find this book to be of great use when dealing with this difficult forensic situation.

Judith H. Gold, M.D., F.R.C.P.(C)
Series Editor,
Clinical Practice Series

Foreword

Juvenile homicide often finds its way on to the front pages of the newspapers. This is especially true for cases of intrafamilial homicide. Thorough scientific reviews of the pertinent issues, however, have been rare in the professional literature. Instead, there have been repetitive publications of individual case reports. What is called for now is an attempt at empirical and scientific examination. Such an approach requires an ordering of the phenomena into some meaningful array so that scientifically valid comparisons can be made. This volume makes considerable strides in this direction by gathering the work of a select group of experts for a much-needed examination of children and adolescents who kill.

The book is divided into two parts: the first deals with clinical issues, and the second addresses forensic and dispositional questions. The first section of the book not only covers the literature with great thoroughness but also reviews the clinical presentation of youthful murderers. Research on this subject tends to be based on samples of small size, and as a result, distinctions among young people who kill may be obscured. Fortunately, some of the findings presented in this section of the book are based on a large sample of cases.

In Chapter 1 Dr. Cornell rejects attempts to characterize *the* juvenile murderer. He appropriately considers juvenile homicide to be a social and legal construct, not a scientific one. Most importantly, Dr. Cornell addresses the question of the cause of juvenile homicide by reframing the issue into the more appropriate and useful query: What are the *various* causes that contribute to a homicide occurring?

Chapters 2 and 3 present data from a study conducted by staff of the Michigan Center for Forensic Psychiatry. The authors describe a group of adolescents arrested for homicide and offer a typology, i.e., an ordering, of juvenile homicide offenders. They suggest that youngsters who kill may be divided into three groups that are distinguishable clinically and factually, but are not, unfortunately, entirely mutually exclusive. They describe three general categories based on the perpetrator's mental state and the circumstances of the offense: first, youth who are psychotic at the time of the offense; second, youth who commit homicide in association with another crime, for example, rape or robbery; and third, youth who commit homicide in association with an interpersonal conflict with the victim, such as intrafamilial homicide and murder of a peer.

Even the most casual student will agree that a murder committed in the course of a gang war is different from the murder of a father by his son or of a brother by his sister. The delineation of youthful murderers into categories that are distinguishable on other than a subjective basis allows further study of the interrelationship of personality, circumstance, and biology in understanding these violent crimes. The Michigan team compared psychotic youthful murderers with the other two groups and found that psychotic offenders, as might be expected, were more likely to have psychiatric histories but less likely to have engaged in criminal activity. In the nonpsychotic homicide group, those who murdered in the course of some other criminal activity had more problems with school adjustment, criminal activity, and substance abuse, but had fewer stressful life events before the offense than those who murdered as a result of interpersonal conflict.

The Michigan observations are consistent with my experience with adolescent youngsters who commit matricide (Mack et al. 1973; Scherl and Mack 1966). In work with a small sample of adolescent boys who killed their mothers, my colleagues and I found the boys to be nonpsychotic but to have a history of serious family dysfunction and conflict. They did not have a history of significant prior criminal activity. For these boys, murder was the culmination of a lifelong history of highly charged family relationships, with feelings severely contained within the family, and an absence of opportunities for emotional discharge outside the home. This was combined with a set of chance circumstances and a failure on the part of society to intervene when it might have.

The first section of the book concludes with an important contribution regarding the adolescent witness to homicide and the concerns that the clinician must have with regard to the adolescent's responses to witnessing lethal violence.

The second section of the book deals with forensic and dispositional matters. In this section, the authors offer guidance for the clinician as he or she proceeds through the criminal justice system. There are useful hints and guidelines with regard to forensic examination of juveniles, matters of competency to stand trial, and criminal responsibility, as well as a longitudinal review of what happens to juvenile homicide offenders from both a legal and a dispositional point of view.

This useful volume makes it clear that there are many forms of juvenile homicide. A school yard killing is not the same as matricide. Murder is often an act with many precedent circumstances, including individual biology, family and personal history, specific precipitating events, and opportunity. The psychiatrist is interested in preventive and causative factors on the one hand and in matters of diagnosis and treatment on the other. The role of the psychiatrist in court and the intersection between psychiatry and the criminal justice system are covered in this volume.

We still need to understand far more clearly, however, what the psychological structure is that *permits* one person to murder another and what psychological admixture provides the energy for it to happen. This volume includes papers that advance our understanding and offer valuable guidelines for further scientific progress in the future.

Donald J. Scherl, M.D.

References

Mack JE, Scherl DJ, Macht LB: Children who kill their mothers, in The Child in His Family: The Impact of Disease and Death. Edited by Anthony EJ, Koupernik C. New York, Wiley Interscience, 1973

Scherl DJ, Mack JE: A study of adolescent matricide. Child Psychiatry 5:569–593, 1966

Acknowledgments

Many individuals have contributed to the completion of this book. First and foremost, we wish to thank our friends and colleagues on the staff of the Center for Forensic Psychiatry in Ann Arbor, Michigan. Our work on juvenile homicide grows out of our clinical experiences, and those of our Center colleagues, in conducting forensic evaluations for Michigan courts. Together we have worked with hundreds of troubled and violent youth, including the adolescent homicide defendants who are the subjects of the research we report here. Our research could not have been possible were it not for the skillful, thorough clinical work of the mental health professionals at the Forensic Center. We appreciate the support of the Center Director, William Meyer, J.D., the Medical Director, Lynn Blunt, M.D., and the former Director of Psychology, Russell Petrella, Ph.D.

A series of individuals have assisted in our research efforts over the past four years. David Benedek helped to initiate our project, from its early planning stages through collection of our "first wave" of data and presentation of our preliminary findings. Special thanks is owed to Lois Staresina, who has assumed a lead role in our ongoing research, serving as a crucial liaison with Michigan courts, and operating our data collection activities. She more than anyone else has made it possible for us to gain the cooperation of so many legal agencies and offices despite so politically sensitive a topic as juvenile crime.

We thank graduate students Susan Paulson of Michigan State University and Peggy Mitchell and Michele Cooley, both of the University of Virginia, for research assistance. We thank Wayne Osgood, Ph.D., now with the University of Nebraska, for statistical consultation and advice.

Our continuing thanks goes to the administrative and support staff of the Forensic Center, especially Linda Collins and Debbie Frederick, for their patience, organizational support, and assistance in so many ways over the years. We wish to thank Jim Romans and Susan Eastman for assistance in obtaining computer records. We should also note the assistance of Cathi Dixon, Steve Hackett, Dawn Bowler, and many others too numerous to mention.

We appreciate the encouragement and advice of Carol Mowbray, Ph.D., as Director, Research and Evaluation Division, for the Michigan Department of Mental Health. Our research has been supported by a series of grants from the Michigan Department of Mental Health.

Finally, we thank our families for emotional support, exceptional patience, and loving encouragement through our labors on this project.

Causes of Juvenile Homicide: A Review of the Literature

DEWEY G. CORNELL, Ph.D.

Chapter 1

Causes of Juvenile Homicide: A Review of the Literature

Over 50 years of published reports have presented widely varying views of the juvenile murderer (Adams 1974; Haizlip et al. 1984). Because juvenile homicide is relatively rare, case studies and reports of small samples are predominant in the literature. For almost any research area, anecdotal or clinical case reports naturally precede studies with larger samples and designs that test specific hypotheses, but this stage seems to have been unusually protracted when it comes to the study of juvenile homicide.

Unfortunately, the case literature on juvenile homicide has not led toward a consolidated perspective. Schmideberg (1973) reports a series of especially callous statements and brutal behavior by youths that illustrates her contention that some juvenile murderers are simply cold-blooded killers who have no concern for human life and feel no guilt for their actions. In contrast, Gardiner (1985) presents extremely sympathetic characterizations of juveniles whose murders seem understandable in light of their abusive upbringing and history of traumatic experiences.

Case studies of juvenile homicide have a strong sensational appeal, even when this is not the author's primary intention. As Thornton and Pray (1975) commented in introducing their case report, "We are presenting the portrait of an impulsive and paranoid young murderer. The intention is not to add to what we feel is already an overemphasized and highly dramatized subject" (p. 176).

Other scholars have succumbed to the evocative nature of the topic and written popular accounts that dramatize the frightening, gruesome, or pathetic aspects of these youth. The criminologist Reinhardt (1970) compiled 17 brief case histories of some exceptionally bizarre and brutal young murderers, who together killed over 41 individuals, including several entire families. Entitled *Nothing Left But ... Murder*, the book has a cover depicting splattered blood and is described in this way by another researcher in the Foreword:

> Dr. Reinhardt parades before the reader a macabre line of young murderers, whose shocking crimes excite the deepest feelings of loathing, anger, and pity.... Hereditary defects, physical injuries, mental aberrations, broken homes, illegitimacy, parental rejection and neglect, grinding poverty, brutalizing sordidness and squalor, festering hatred and pent-up rage, and other such corrosive influences weave in and out and play upon the lives of the killers, relentlessly destroying them until, in the words of Dr. Reinhardt, there was "nothing left but murder." (p. ix)

The provocative nature of the topic seems to have inspired a wide range of speculation, even in research reports. For example, one author (Sorrells 1977) categorized his sample of adolescent murderers by astrological sign, which he reported was done at his secretary's suggestion. Although no significance testing was presented, he notes that 8 of 37 cases were Scorpios and wonders if there might be "something special" about those born under this sign!

The Search for Causal Explanations

The fields of psychology and psychiatry are far from determining formal scientific answers to causal questions about violent behavior in general, much less juvenile homicide in particular. However, juvenile homicide is such a provocative phenomenon that it naturally stimulates great interest in questions of causation. Why did this happen? How could someone so young come to commit murder? Was there something in the youth's background or personality that could explain what happened? Clinicians face such causal questions whenever they evaluate a juvenile charged with murder. Even if not explicit, they are implicit in most referrals. Certainly the clinician preparing to testify as an expert witness should be prepared to field these very difficult questions.

It follows that the search for causal factors in juvenile homicide may be driven as much by social and legal concerns as scientific ones. However, most questions about the "cause" of juvenile homicide are too broad and poorly specified to be meaningful. The question, "What is the cause of juvenile homicide?" can be answered from many different perspectives or levels of analysis, which are not mutually exclusive. Social, psychological, and biological factors all may contribute to violent behavior (Crowell et al. 1987; Grinker 1971; Keith 1984).

Despite general recognition of the multiplicity of causal factors in human behavior, even formal, scientific discussions of causality are clouded by ambiguous language:

> We all tend to frame every sort of idea of determination, as well as every kind of explanation, in a causal *language* that often distorts the meaning we really wish to convey. Thus we usually cover the concepts of origin, ground, motive, and even reason with the single word "cause"; and we readily confuse logical entailment with causation, and logical consequence with effect. (Bunge 1979, p. 346)

Legal concepts of cause are no clearer than scientific ones, because the law explicitly endorses "common sense" principles of causality (Hart and Honoré 1985). Common sense is extraordinarily vague, inconsistent, and idiosyncratic when it comes to causal thinking. Often the "cause" of an event is simply assumed to be whatever is unique or unusual about its circumstances. In actuality, any event is the product of a multiplicity of factors, and what is termed causal is often a matter of perspective.

Consider the simple example of an automobile accident that occurred when Jack Jones was speeding through an intersection and struck an oncoming car driven by Jane Jones, who was attempting to turn across his path. Many factors could be said to have "caused" the accident, depending on the frame of reference and type of causal question being asked. A police officer might view this intersection as a scene of many accidents *because* there was no traffic signal to permit turning, or *because* visibility from the intersection was poor due to a curve in the road.

In contrast, an automobile safety engineer might observe that the poor brakes in Jack's car, combined with slick road conditions, prevented his car from stopping in time. From an altogether different frame of reference, Jack Jones could be said to have caused the accident because he was driving too fast; or perhaps Jane Jones used poor judgment in pulling across his path. From a motivational point of view, Jack was speeding *because* he was late for work, and Jane neglected to use good judgment *because* she was preoccupied with a recent marital argument.

Finally, Jack's psychoanalyst suggested that Jack struck the car *because* it was driven by his wife and he was expressing unconscious hostility toward her. Jane's psychoanalyst saw the accident as another example of her tendency to let Jack "run over" her in their marriage.

Sociological approaches to juvenile violence address factors somewhat analogous to that of the policeman who has seen one accident after another in the same intersection and draws causal conclusions about the circumstances under which accidents take place. Similarly, psychobiologically oriented investigators may be likened to the safety engineer in their emphasis on physical dysfunction and operational factors. Such analogies are admittedly crude and imperfect, but they illustrate a general point. The vague usage of the term "cause" in everyday language has carried over into social science discourse and greatly complicates behavioral research. Unfortunately, there can be no resolution of many controversies until there is a generally agreed-upon taxonomy to define the different meanings of the term "cause" when applied to human behavior.

Incidence of Juvenile Homicide

Juvenile homicide represents only a fraction of all juvenile crime and a small percentage of all homicides. The Uniform Crime Reports published each year by the FBI present the number of individuals in different age groups arrested for various index offenses. In 1986, juveniles (under age 18) made up 16.8 percent of all 10,392,177 persons reported arrested around the nation. Juveniles constituted 33.5 percent of all persons arrested for property crime, but only 15.4 percent of all persons arrested for violent crime (Federal Bureau of Investigation 1978–87).

The proportion of juvenile arrests for homicide is even lower. The 1,396 juveniles arrested for murder or nonnegligent homicide in 1986 represented only about 8.7 percent of the total arrested nationwide. For the 10-year period 1977–1986, the proportion of murders (including nonnegligent homicide) committed by juveniles has ranged from a low of 7.3 percent in 1984 to a high of 9.7 percent in 1977 (Federal Bureau of Investigation 1978–87).

The incidence of juvenile homicide increases markedly through the adolescent years. In 1986, only 12 children age 12 or under were arrested for homicide, but the numbers increased steadily to 134 13- to 14-year-olds, 245 15-year-olds, 443 16-year-olds, and 552 17-year-olds. As indicated in Figure 1, age differences have remained relatively stable over time.

Data in Figure 1 are actual arrest frequencies and are not corrected for differences in the underlying population size at each age level. An approximation of the juvenile homicide arrest *rate* can be determined by dividing the number arrested by the underlying population size for the same age group. Figure 2

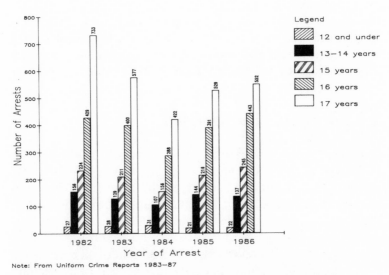

FIGURE 1. Ages of U.S. juveniles arrested for homicide 1982–1986.

presents the homicide rate for juveniles (here defined as youths aged 10 through 17) compared with that for adults (ages 18 and older) for the 10-year period 1977–1986.

Figure 2 reveals that the annual arrest rate for juveniles is approximately half that for adults, typically 8 to 10 adults per 100,000 adults, but only about 3 to 5 juveniles per 100,000 juveniles. The two rates appear to fluctuate together over the years, suggesting that whatever factors affect the homicide arrest rate similarly affect adults and juveniles. The correlation between the two arrest rates for the 10-year period is quite large, approximately 0.81.

Data in Figure 2 are derived from combining information from Uniform Crime Reports and U.S. Census Bureau reports (Bureau of the Census 1982, 1987). Because these reports use different data sources and because arrest figures are based only on reporting agencies, the rates presented here should be regarded as rough estimates. The population size for juveniles is limited to ages 10 through 17 years because the incidence of homicide arrests for children under age 10 is negligible relative

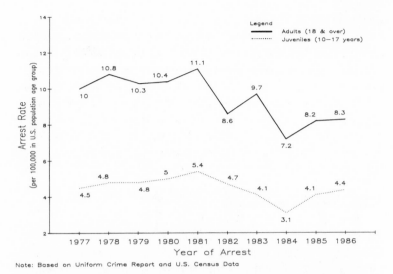

FIGURE 2. U.S. juvenile and adult homicide arrest rates 1977–1986.

to the size of the underlying population (99 reported arrests in 10 years). (In addition, homicides committed by young children may not result in arrests and would not be reported in the Uniform Crime Reports.)

More detailed information about the victims and circumstances of juvenile homicides across the nation are available. Rowley et al. (1987) report a secondary analysis of juvenile homicide data contained in the Supplementary Homicide Report of the 1985 Uniform Crime Report. For the 787 juveniles (ages 10 to 17) arrested for murder or nonnegligent manslaughter in 1984, 687 (93 percent) were male and 429 (73 percent) were classified as white. Data reported for the relationship between juvenile and victim indicate that approximately half (49 percent) of the victims were acquaintances, approximately one-third (33 percent) were strangers, and the remainder (18 percent) were family members. About half (65 of 139, or 47 percent) of the family member victims were parents or stepparents.

The data summarized by Rowley and colleagues are par-

9

ticularly useful because they constitute a nationwide sample not subject to the potential referral biases of clinical samples reported in the literature. For example, the attention given to juveniles who murder parents is clearly disproportionate to other, much more common, forms of juvenile homicide. The smaller the sample, the more disproportionate the attention to unusual cases. Clinical formulations based on more sensational or high-profile cases such as parricide may not apply to the wider group of juveniles who engage in homicidally violent behavior.

Major Psychopathology

The association between juvenile homicide and major psychopathology has been explored by numerous authors. A recurrent assumption of this work is that it is so abnormal for a juvenile to commit homicide that some form of major psychopathology *must* be present. In an influential clinical article, Easson and Steinhilber (1961) articulated this view:

> In many studies on homicide there are murderers designated as "normal" psychologically and there are murders classified as being "without motive," often by these same "normal" people. With these designations we would disagree. In our culture, "normal" people do not commit murder. No murder is "without motive." These classifications are most often seen in descriptions of murders by children and young adults. More intensive investigation, in most circumstances impossible owing to the circumstances of the investigation, would, we believe, have given indication of underlying psychopathology in these cases. (p. 28)

Variability in diagnostic terminology and diagnostic criteria make comparisons across studies difficult. Consequently, the findings of the following studies will be presented using the diagnostic terms employed by the authors.

Lauretta Bender (Bender 1959; Bender and Curran 1940; Bender et al. 1937) was one of the earliest authorities to emphasize the role of psychotic processes in juvenile homicide. She presented clinical data on 33 youths she had examined in the course of approximately 24 years of clinical work. Fourteen of the cases involved accidental or unintended homicide, so that only 19 actually committed intentional homicide.

Bender (1959) maintained that schizophrenia, brain disease, or epilepsy was present in all but three youths who committed intentional homicide. In particular, she contended that "pseudopsychopathic defenses may mask the basic schizophrenic picture or organic or epileptic disorganization for a while" (p. 512). Several youths not viewed as psychotic at the time of court hearing subsequently became psychotic and had to be transferred from correctional facilities to hospitals.

Bender's stature in the field gave strong support to the hypothesis that homicidally violent youth might suffer from latent or incipient psychosis that otherwise might be overlooked. Nevertheless, generalizations from the Bender cases must be made with caution, given the selective nature of the sample (clinically referred subjects) and the diagnostic criteria in use at the time. Many authors who have cited Bender's work fail to note the highly selective nature of the sample.

In contrast, another early report that found little evidence of major psychopathology went relatively unnoticed. Patterson (1943) presented six cases in which a young male (age range 11–14) killed a family member or peer. None of these youths were diagnosed as suffering from major psychopathology, although one was mildly retarded. Patterson emphasized the impact of unstable and emotionally unsupportive families that impair the normal development of inhibitions against aggression.

Two other reports emphasized highly unusual cases. Wittman and Astrachan (1949) described a highly intelligent, seemingly well-adjusted, 18-year-old University of Chicago student who murdered two women and a child during a series of midnight burglaries. The youth claimed amnesia for the offenses and identified another self he called "6" who carried out the crimes. The authors ruled out malingering, psychosis, and psy-

11

chopathic personality and concluded that the youth suffered from hysterical fugue states.

Medlicott (1955) reported a most unusual case of two adolescent girls who suffered "paranoia of the exalted type in a setting of *folie à deux.*" The two brutally murdered one of their mothers who threatened them with separation. They both suffered from severe mood swings and shared grandiose delusions of their supernatural abilities, religious insights, and artistic genius. Follow-up information by Medlicott (cited in Cormier and Markus 1980) indicates that the women clinically improved and were released within five years. One became a schoolteacher, and the other became an airline hostess.

In one of the few studies to move beyond a case study approach, Sendi and Blomgren (1975) studied 10 adolescents who had been admitted to a state psychiatric hospital after committing homicide and compared them to 10 adolescents who had merely attempted homicide, as well as to 10 psychiatric controls who had not engaged in homicidal behavior. They found that 6 of 10 adolescents who had committed homicide were diagnosed as schizophrenic (the remaining 4 were diagnosed as personality disordered), compared with only 3 of 10 who had attempted homicide and 4 of 10 nonhomicidal controls. This represents a very marginal difference in incidence of schizophrenia and probably is affected by subject selection factors that would identify the most disturbed cases.

A number of reports further document the range of diagnoses that have been applied to juvenile homicide cases. Russell (1965, 1973, 1979) has issued a series of reports on an accumulating number of cases he has studied over a 15-year period. Of 24 cases, Russell diagnosed the youths as follows: neurotic (13 cases), antisocial (3 cases), schizoid (5 cases), and schizophrenic (2 cases). Two more were diagnosed as suffering from what he termed a syndrome of severe childhood narcissism (Russell 1979).

Malmquist (1971) evaluated 20 court-referred youths and diagnosed depressive disorders (10 cases), personality disorders (7), and schizophrenia (3). Rosner et al. (1979) reviewed clinical records of 45 adolescents (age range, 16–18) evaluated at an urban New York forensic clinic between 1970 and 1974. Diagnoses were as follows: personality disorder (22 cases), schizophrenia (10), transient situation disturbances (5), no mental disorder (4), and diagnosis deferred (4).

Yates et al. (1984) compared 46 young males (mean age 18.4) convicted of murder with 262 males convicted of other violent crimes against a person, as well as with 31 males convicted of property offenses. Subjects were youths remanded to a California Youth Authority training school. In the entire sample, only two subjects were diagnosed as having an organic disorder and only three were diagnosed as schizophrenic. The most prevalent diagnoses among the murderers were personality disorder (34.8 percent) and conduct disorder (30.4 percent).

Other authors did not report detailed diagnostic information on their subjects, but did rule out psychosis. In that group are included 4 cases reported by Stearns (1957); 5 cases in Finland described by Hellsten and Katila (1965); 8 of 9 cases studied by King (1975); 11 cases collected in England and Wales by Walshe-Brennan (1976, 1977); the "majority" of 30 cases reviewed by Corder et al. (1976); and 31 cases surveyed by Sorrells (1977, 1980). Sorrells (1980) later suggested that some of his subjects might be classified "prepsychotic" because of their lack of relationships with others and the extreme callousness of their behavior. However, he reported no overt psychotic symptoms and no follow-up information to support this prediction.

Adopting a different methodological approach and emphasis, Lewis et al. (1985) reported background characteristics of nine males who were clinically evaluated during adolescence (ages 12 to 18) and *later* committed homicide (ages 15 to 26). The authors note that records of the prehomicide evaluation indicate that *all* of the subjects had a history of psychotic symptoms, as well as a first-degree relative with reported psychotic symptoms or psychiatric hospitalization. All nine subjects had a history of serious violence and nearly all had a history of physical abuse. Lewis and colleagues also reported

13

that almost all had indications of major neurological impairment. These nine subjects were compared to 24 incarcerated delinquents from another clinical study who as of six years later had no state record of arrests for serious felonies. They found that the best discriminator between groups was the presence of a combination of neuropsychiatric impairment, parental psychosis, physical abuse, and prior violent behavior.

It is difficult to assess the general applicability of the findings of Lewis et al. (1985), given the small and selective nature of the samples, but the study of youths who were evaluated before committing homicide may be a useful research strategy. The ability to identify even a small subgroup of homicidally violent youths would be a significant advance.

Episodic Dyscontrol or Brief Psychosis

The apparent lack of overt psychopathology in many murderers is particularly troubling when no clear motive or justification for the homicide is evident (Menninger and Mayman 1956; Satten et al. 1960; Smith 1965; Stearns 1957). When a perpetrator acts in an especially impulsive, brutal manner and afterwards cannot (or will not) recall the act, the clinician is hard-pressed to explain the event. This problem was addressed by Menninger and Mayman (1956) when they proposed a new diagnostic phenomenon, *episodic dyscontrol*. Episodic dyscontrol was defined as a syndrome in which an individual with severe ego developmental deficits experiences episodes of severe loss of impulse control.

Episodic dyscontrol has been hypothesized as a factor in several case reports (McCarthy 1978; Miller and Looney 1974; Satten et al. 1960; Smith 1965). Sadoff (1971) described two cases of homicide in which he contended that both perpetrators (who murdered abusive parents) manifested a borderline or schizoid personality, and that they suffered an "acute paranoid schizophrenic reaction which remitted spontaneously" (p. 68).

14

It seems tenuous to diagnose psychosis because of the impulsivity and rage of the perpetrator at the time of the homicide. There should be some evidence of delusions, hallucinations, formal thought disorder, or grossly bizarre behavior to support a diagnosis of psychosis. Although one might contend that homicide represents bizarre or irrational behavior in itself, this reasoning would imply that homicide is always a psychotic act and would apply essentially to all acts of impulsive violence.

Even in subjects diagnosed with borderline personality disorder, the presence of clear-cut psychotic episodes is unusual and subject to question (Pope et al. 1985). The borderline patient who claims psychotic symptoms demands close diagnostic scrutiny, because such claims may be exaggerated or presented for self-serving purposes.

The tendency of some clinicians to overdiagnose psychosis in cases of adolescent homicide is illustrated by three cases of matricide presented by Mohr and McKnight (1971). All three youths (ages 15–17) were diagnosed schizophrenic and found not guilty by reason of insanity, essentially because of the brutality and apparent senselessness of the crimes. The murders were premeditated ambushes with no apparent precipitants. None of the youths exhibited psychotic symptoms at any time before the murder or during several years of hospitalization that followed. Two were released and reported to be doing well, and the third was kept in the hospital solely because of concerns about his "manipulative character disorder" (p. 31).

Although acknowledging that the adolescents he examined presented no evidence of psychosis before or after the murder, even on psychological testing, Smith (1965) contended that their claimed amnesia for the offense was symptomatic of regression to the primitive, psychotic level of ego functioning that constituted episodic dyscontrol. The use of partial or complete amnesia as a basis for the diagnosis of psychosis seems unjustified. Many criminal defendants claim poor memory for their behavior (Schacter 1986). Such claims may reflect an attempt to disown responsibility for the act, to avoid further questioning, or to appear mentally disturbed. The layperson defendant may assume that amnesia is a common symptom of severe mental disorder, adding it to a malingered presentation.

Experienced forensic clinicians who have had the repeated experience of interviewing defendants who at first report amnesia, but later recant and acknowledge complete memory for their offense, quickly become skeptical of claimed amnesia. The difficulty of distinguishing genuine from malingered amnesia is well known (Rogers 1986; Schacter 1986), so that clinicians should be reluctant to reach firm diagnostic conclusions on the basis of claimed amnesia.

Even genuine amnesia offers poor support for a psychotic diagnosis. Amnesia does not in itself imply that a person's behavior during the forgotten time period was in any way less intentional or rational (Rogers 1986; Schacter 1986). Many individuals suffer poor or incomplete memory for traumatic or terrifying events, or for periods when they acted impulsively in a state of intense emotional arousal.

Brain Dysfunction

A recurrent hypothesis in the literature is that homicidal behavior in juveniles is the product of brain damage. Lewis (1981) has championed the position that homicidally aggressive youths should receive comprehensive neuropsychiatric examinations because of a reported high incidence of both "hard" and "soft" signs of neurological abnormalities. However, the evidence remains equivocal and the ideas controversial.

In Bender's sample of 33 cases described earlier (Bender 1959), 10 of 15 available EEGs were abnormal and suggested epilepsy, although apparently only three subjects were diagnosed epileptic.

Michaels (1961) commented that in six of eight cases reported by Easson and Steinhilber (1961) the subjects had histories of persistent enuresis until age six or seven and that three of eight had seizure disorders. He argued that such findings among these and other delinquent youth indicate a "psychosomatic disposition" (p. 491) toward violence, which was linked to personality characteristics such as irritability, explosive temper, and poor ability to inhibit or control impulses. Woods (1961) went so far as to claim that a specific EEG abnormal dysrhythmia consisting of positive spiking at the rate of 6 and 14 per second was associated with episodes of homicidally violent behavior in youth.

Sendi and Blomgren (1975) found that a diagnosis of organic brain syndrome actually occurred more frequently in hospitalized adolescents who had *attempted* homicide (7 of 10 cases) than in adolescents who had *committed* homicide (0 of 10 with an organic diagnosis). Walshe-Brennan (1977) investigated records of 11 youths (ages 10–15) who committed homicide in England and Wales from 1957 to 1972. Nothing abnormal was found on routine exams, which included x-rays of the skull and EEGs.

The absence of neurological findings cannot simply be attributed to inadequate evaluation (see Easson and Steinhilber 1961; Greenberg and Blank 1970; Scherl and Mack 1966; Welshe-Brennan 1977). For example, Scherl and Mack (1966) reported that extensive neurological investigation, including four EEGs, skull films, a lumbar puncture, and psychological testing, revealed no organic pathology in a 14-year-old who murdered his psychologically abusive mother. The youth was treated with psychotherapy in a hospital setting over a period of years and was diagnosed as suffering from a character disorder.

Although King (1975) approached the issue of cognitive deficits from a social-ecological perspective, his analysis provides a useful framework for understanding the behavioral implications of neuropsychological impairment. He stressed that the educational and language deficiencies of violent youth severely limit their ability to resolve interpersonal conflicts and interact appropriately with others. Aggressive behavior represents one of the few available alternatives for youths who cannot use verbal reasoning or verbal communication skills to cope with the frustrations and problems of daily life.

General intellectual deficits in juvenile murderers have been noted. Hays et al. (1978) examined IQ data from the Wechsler Intelligence Scale for Children (WISC) for 25 juvenile murderers (ages 15–16) and 39 status offenders. The mean full scale IQ for the murderers was 80.0, significantly lower than the mean IQ of 87.1 for the status offenders. In addition, verbal IQs were significantly lower (by 4 to 6 points) than performance IQs for both groups.

Lewis et al. (1981) reported results of neuropsychiatric evaluations of 97 incarcerated juvenile delinquents, nearly all of whom had a history of violent behavior. Contrasting more violent subjects to less violent subjects (on the basis of a global rating scale), the authors found that the more violent delinquents were more paranoid, were more loose and illogical in their speech, and more often manifested at least one major sign of neurological dysfunction. In addition, they were more likely to have been abused and to have witnessed extreme violence. No differences in the incidence of EEG abnormalities were found. Lewis and colleagues noted the existence of possible bias in their findings because the clinical examiners were not blind to the identities of the most violent subjects.

Finally, it must be noted that a well-documented association between homicide and neuropsychiatric symptoms would be only the beginning step in examining the causal relationship between brain dysfunction and aggressive behavior. Proponents of social theories might contend that juvenile violence and problems such as perinatal difficulties are *both* consequences of low socioeconomic status. Others might argue that a history of head injury reflects preexisting impulsiveness and a predisposition to dangerous, violent behavior. As always, it is important to make use of appropriate control groups (for example, nonviolent delinquents matched on socioeconomic variables).

Intrafamilial Homicide

Sargent (1962) presented the classic hypothesis that "sometimes the child who kills is acting as the unwitting lethal agent of an adult (usually a parent) who unconsciously prompts the child to kill so that he can vicariously enjoy the benefits of the act" (p. 35). He contended that the adult takes advantage of the child's immaturity and emotional dependency to inflame any preexisting hostility that the child has toward the victim. Sargent presented five case examples to illustrate the phenomenon. These include several youths who murdered an abusive parent or stepparent with the implicit or even explicit support of the spouse. In a later report of two more cases, Sargent (1971) elaborated on the sometimes subtle ways in which the message to kill was transmitted from adult to child.

Sargent suggested that when a juvenile murders under the influence of an adult, it should constitute extenuating circumstances that diminish the youth's responsibility for the crime. A similar view (Mones 1985) was proposed by an attorney who reviewed records on seven teenagers who committed parricide. He noted that in all but one case the youths had no history of delinquency and that they all suffered some form of physical or psychological abuse. He compared their plight to that of an abused spouse who is unable to flee the abusive relationship and resorts to murder. Similar ideas are reflected in a collection of cases compiled by a *Time* magazine writer (Morris 1985).

The literature contains ample case examples of youths who committed homicide in response to an abusive family member (Cormier et al. 1978; Duncan and Duncan 1971; Kalogerakis 1971; Mohr and McKnight 1971; Post 1982; Sadoff 1971; Tanay 1973, 1976). Mohr and McKnight (1971) used the term "lockage phenomenon" to refer to the intense interpersonal relationship between the youth and family member prior to the homicide. The youth is described as locked into a highly conflictual, dependent relationship that he or she can no longer sustain or give up.

Duncan and Duncan (1971), as well as Post (1982), emphasized the role of situational factors, such as the availability of weapons and the use of drugs, which help precipitate violence in a chronically abusive relationship. Tanay (1973, 1976) contended that "reactive parricide" constitutes a particular form of homicide in which the youth responds to severe family conflicts. Remarkably, Tanay suggested that reactive parricide has a *beneficial* effect on both the perpetrator and surviving family members, because they are freed from the abusive parent.

The overwhelming majority of juvenile murderers are male, so that very little has been written about females. Anthony and Rizzo (1973) report cases of two 15-year-old girls, one who killed, and one who attempted to kill, her father. In both cases, the homicides represented the culmination of years of extreme psychological abuse. In the first case, the father had sexually abused three daughters and a son over a period of years and even murdered a newborn produced from one of the incestuous encounters.

Corder et al. (1976) conducted one of the few empirical studies of adolescents who committed parricide, comparing 10 such cases to 10 who murdered another relative or close acquaintance and 10 who murdered a stranger. Corder and colleagues found that the 30 youths as a whole had a high incidence of family maladjustment (marital conflict, child abuse, parent substance abuse and criminal activity, and so forth). The most consistent differences were between adolescents who murdered parents and those who murdered strangers. The adolescents who committed parricide were less likely to have a history of poor impulse control and aggressive behavior, or prior placement in a juvenile facility. They were more likely to be described as overly attached to their mother and sexually overstimulated by her, but less likely to have had dating relationships with peers. They were less likely to have planned the murder and more likely to claim amnesia for the act.

20

Psychodynamic Factors

Smith (1965) examined eight adolescents (ages 14–21) in developing his theory that adolescent murderers suffer from impaired ego development due to early oral deprivation associated with an unstable family environment. He elaborated upon the earlier concept of episodic dyscontrol (Menninger and Mayman 1956), speculating that rageful episodes served a defensive function of preventing a more extensive disintegration of the personality.

Scherl and Mack (1966) reported that three cases of adolescent matricide had in common a psychologically abusive, dominating mother and a passive, uninvolved father. Later, Mack et al. (1973) emphasized the role of oedipal and dependency conflicts in juveniles who murdered their mothers. Drawing upon mythology and literature, as well as a variety of case studies, they present the thesis that victims of matricide induced intolerable intrapsychic conflicts in their sons by their sexually provocative behavior, which ranged from flagrant marital infidelity to overtly incestuous behavior. They note that matricide can be viewed as the "primal crime" because the child's first experiences of hostility toward others take place in the context of the maternal relationship.

Malmquist (1971) searched for "premonitory factors" among 20 youths he had personally evaluated for legal purposes. He emphasized factors typically associated with depression, hypothesizing that homicidal aggression constituted a displacement from anger at self. He described homicidal youths as exhibiting a behavior change involving intense brooding, pessimism, and self-criticism, accompanied by muted or indirect calls for help from others.

Miller and Looney (1974) discussed the prediction of adolescent homicide from a psychoanalytic perspective, based on clinical study of 10 cases. Surprisingly, the authors claimed to have "predicted murder in advance of a homicidal attempt in all but two of the cases studied" (p. 190). They postulate that the predisposition to murder is determined by the aggressor's potential for "dehumanizing" the victim. Dehumanization is described as the perception of a person as merely a frustrating object rather than a human being with whom one can identify and empathize. Dehumanization may occur to varying degrees or on an episodic basis and is seen developmentally in young children when they occasionally become enraged.

Miller and Looney contend that the high-risk murderers who totally dehumanize others are "primitive, narcissistic, and omnipotent personalities who show both a disinclination to value human life and an ego-syntonic acceptance of violence" (p. 192). In contrast, other murderers only dehumanize during periods of episodic dyscontrol and act in response to mixed sexual and aggressive conflict. The authors' claims for the predictive validity of this approach seem overstated and unsubstantiated. Nevertheless, the concept of dehumanization seems useful and suggests the potential value of assessing violent youths from an object relations framework. Dehumanization may reflect a general means of overcoming the normal inhibitions against violent behavior. For example, in time of war soldiers may develop dehumanizing attitudes (often in response to specific propaganda) that the enemy is inhuman or animalistic.

McCarthy (1978) built upon concepts of dehumanization and episodic dyscontrol in elaborating a theory of narcissistic deficits in homicidal youth. Based on a review of clinical and psychological test data on 10 hospitalized adolescents who had committed murder, McCarthy concluded that "homicidal rage can be understood as an attempt at reparation of the self. Its expression affirmed a sense of reality and restored infantile omnipotence" (p. 25).

Preadolescent Homicidal Behavior

There have been few attempts to study homicidal behavior in young children, largely because it is so rare, or at least rarely reported. For example, Uniform Crime Report (Federal Bureau of Investigation 1987) figures indicate that only 7 children under age 10 (and only 15 between the ages of 10 and 12) were arrested for homicide in 1986. In contrast, 4201 children under age 10 were arrested for burglary and 15,238 were arrested for larceny or theft.

Homicide committed by preadolescent children may be qualitatively different than homicide committed by adolescents for a number of reasons. Young children have a very limited understanding of death, and their aggressive behavior may be more impulsive and less goal-directed than in adolescence. Legally, they are considered less responsible for their actions and typically they are immune from prosecution.

Carek and Watson (1964) reported the case of a 10-year-old boy who was left to babysit five younger siblings. When his two younger brothers became defiant, he retrieved his father's loaded shotgun and threatened them. After one of the brothers teasingly dropped a toy down the gun barrel, the oldest boy angrily pulled the trigger, killing his brother. At first the family attempted to deny the murder and described it as an accident. However, both parents and the boy developed multiple symptoms, including feelings of anxiety, preoccupation, and depression. Carek and Watson argued for the importance of hospital treatment of the boy, with conjoint treatment of the parents. All parties were exceptionally resistant to treatment, but after five months of hospitalization the boy tearfully described the tragedy in detail and for the first time fully acknowledged that the killing was not an accident. After this disclosure, the boy was able to make progress in psychotherapy, working through his difficult feelings of anger and guilt.

Adelson (1972) described five cases of young children (ages 2½ to 8) who inflicted fatal head injuries on infants under 1 year of age. This represented only 0.005 percent of the 975 homicides investigated by the Cuyahoga County (Ohio) Coroner's Office in a 3½-year period. There was no evidence that the children acted in response to adult influence or that the infants had been abused by others. Adelson commented that these types of cases did not fit the pattern of either family disturbance or individual psychopathology described in previous literature. Instead, the children seem to have acted impulsively and naively in response to the infant's crying by striking or dropping the baby in frustration. In several cases there was suggestion that the child had been jealous of the baby, but the more critical factor seems to be that the children were not adequately supervised.

Paluszny and McNabb (1975) discussed the role of guilt and repression in the treatment of a six-year-old named Maggie who killed her four-month-old brother by fracturing his skull while she was left by her mother to look after him and her two-year-old sister. First seen for outpatient therapy two days afterwards, the girl soon repressed all memory of the event and began to evidence other memory and concentration problems as well. Over the course of play therapy, Maggie was preoccupied with themes of sibling rivalry and death. As her memory of her brother returned, she began to misbehave regularly and seemed to provoke punishment as a means of coping with her guilt. Over 18 months of therapy focused on different aspects of Maggie's conflicts over the death, including feelings of guilt, depression, and anger with her mother.

A somewhat different perspective on child homicide was offered by Tooley (1975), who described two hospitalized six-year-olds who had repeatedly attempted to kill younger siblings by methods that included fire setting, drowning, and poisoning. Both children were described as resourceful, unusually self-assured, verbally precocious, and provocative. In both cases the children appeared to be acting out the unstated wishes of overburdened mothers who were surprisingly complacent about the assaults and clearly favored the older child.

The role of parent influence in the homicidal behavior of young children was further illustrated by Tucker and Cornwall (1977). They reported a case of *folie à deux* involving a 10-year-old boy and his paranoid mother. Over a six-month period the mother convinced her son that his father was attempting to kill them, although both knew that the father lived across the country. Following his mother's plans, the boy flew across country alone and burned his father's house down in the night, the father just escaping with his life. The boy's psychotic features subsided with three months of hospital treatment, and he was discharged to the care of his father and outpatient therapy.

Bernstein (1978) provided a detailed case history of seven-year-old David, who committed premeditated murder by stabbing a female peer on the way home from school. He had a history of fighting and arguing with the girl, but otherwise was not considered a disciplinary problem at home or school. There was a history of chronic marital discord and frequent physical violence in the family, although no definite indication that David was the subject of physical abuse. His neurological evaluation, including EEG, was normal, and there was no indication of psychosis. Initially David was placed in a foster home, and after one year he was hospitalized and treated with psychotherapy. He had problems with lying and teasing, but there was no recurrence of severe violent behavior. David was described as having trouble expressing aggressive feelings and had much fear of retribution for any aggressive behavior he exhibited. He expressed concern for the victim's family, but could never talk about the murder. After three years in the hospital he was felt to be considerably improved and was discharged to outpatient psychotherapy.

Pfeffer (1980) emphasized the importance of hospital treatment for highly assaultive children (ages 6–12), citing five case examples of extremely aggressive children who nearly killed their victims. She associated homicidal aggression in children with attempts to master violent trauma and with severe ego deficits, including mental retardation and psychosis.

There are at least two empirical studies of homicidally aggressive young children, although only one of the subjects actually committed homicide. Petti and Davidman (1981) reported that a group of nine hospitalized children (ages 6 to 11) who had engaged in homicidally aggressive behavior had lower scores on the Children's Locus of Control Scale (reflecting less sense of internal control) than a group of psychiatric controls matched on sex, age, and IQ. Only one child actually commit-ted homicide, and only one child was hospitalized specifically for homicidal behavior.

Lewis and colleagues (Lewis et al. 1983) also examined records of 21 "homicidally aggressive" young children (ages 3 to 12) who had been admitted to a single child psychiatric unit. None of these children actually committed homicide, but all had a history of multiple aggressive acts. The children were compared to 30 child inpatients not classified as homicidally aggressive on a large number of developmental, family, medi-cal, psychiatric, psychological, and educational variables. The authors report that children in the aggressive group were more likely to have had a seizure, but groups did *not* differ on EEG abnormalities, perinatal difficulties, history of head injury, soft neurological signs, hallucinations, or learning disabilities.

Categorization of Juvenile Homicide Offenders

The diversity of juveniles who commit homicide has led sev-eral researchers to propose subgrouping them according to var-ious factors, including the perpetrator-victim relationship and the clinical characteristics of the juvenile (Cormier et al. 1971a; Miller and Looney 1974; Russell 1965; Zenoff and Zients 1979).

As noted above, Corder and colleagues (1976) distin-guished adolescents who murdered parents from those who murdered other relatives or acquaintances and from those who murdered strangers. The most consistent differences were be-tween those who murdered parents and those who murdered strangers, with the other group falling in between on many measures of background characteristics.

Zenoff and Zients (1979) studied 19 youths under age 16 who were charged with murder in the District of Columbia and referred for evaluation by the juvenile court. Based on review of clinical records, they proposed three subgroups. Six males murdered acquaintances impulsively during interpersonal dis-putes and were described as suffering from sexual-identity conflicts but generally lacking a history of delinquent behavior. Seven other youths murdered strangers in the course of a robbery or for no discernible reason. These youths were described as "nonempathic murderers" with little concern for others and a history of school problems, prior assaultive behavior, and property offenses. The remaining seven youths were a heterogeneous group who killed accidentally or in self-defense.

Solway and colleagues (1981) collected psychological test data on 18 adolescent murderers in Texas, distinguishing an "emotionally disturbed" group (12 cases) who murdered relatives or close acquaintances from a "criminal or psychopathic-like" group (6 cases) who murdered either a stranger or distant acquaintance "in the context of some other deviant or criminal behavior" (p. 203). The disturbed group obtained higher scores on the Minnesota Multiphasic Personality Inventory scale 8 and gave more popular responses and total human content on the Rorschach test. The disturbed group also had higher verbal IQs on the Wechsler Intelligence Scale for Children (Revised), whereas the criminal group had higher scores on the performance scales. Other subgroupings of the 18 cases resulted in few significant findings, although the small sample size greatly limited the power of significance tests.

Cornell et al. (1987a, 1987b) emphasized distinguishing among adolescents based on the circumstances of the homicide. They classified 72 youths charged with homicide into three groups: *psychotic*—adolescents who manifested overt psychotic symptoms at the time of the offense; *crime*—adolescents who murdered in the course of another criminal activity such as robbery or rape; and *conflict*—those who were involved in an interpersonal conflict or dispute with the victim. Empirical support for the typology is reviewed in Chapter 3.

Conclusion

What can be learned from the literature that would benefit future researchers and future users of juvenile homicide research? The following observations may be made:

1. Because a wealth of case studies are available, publication of further case reports *outside the context of empirical study* seems unnecessary. The diversity of juvenile murders is clear, and numerous cases can be cited to illustrate a variety of theoretical positions. Much more attention must be paid to sampling issues. Samples derived entirely from the author's clinical practice have already contributed as much to the literature as they probably can. Samples obtained from hospital settings are likely to be highly biased in the direction of major psychopathology, yet such cases appear to represent a minority of all juveniles who commit homicide. Authors of such studies need to be more conservative in their generalizations.

Samples of youths referred by the courts for forensic evaluation can be quite diverse, but many youths are never referred for evaluation. The courts exert a selective influence on which cases are available for study. Court-referred cases may be youths who exhibit strange or unusual behavior suggestive of mental illness, who commit especially brutal or heinous murders, who kill family members, or who have a history of psychological treatment. Cases also may be referred simply because of the youth of the offender or the thoroughness of a defense attorney. Research on court-referred samples should be examined for representativeness, and findings should be replicated on a broader sample whenever possible.

2. The compelling social significance of juvenile homicide should not lead to a lessening of well-accepted methodological standards. Claims of group differences have been made without supporting tests of statistical significance, and the issue of "probability pyramiding" (attaining a small proportion of significant results by chance) is rarely addressed. When researchers rely on chart reviews, interviews, ratings, or similar methods, evidence for the interrater reliability of the measures must be presented. Moreover, it must be explicit whether or not raters are blind to group membership of the subjects they rate.

3. Studies that attempt to characterize *the* juvenile murderer can be rejected automatically as naive. A half-century of

case studies alone has documented the considerable heterogeneity of youths who commit homicidal acts. More recent studies demonstrate important differences *within* homicide groups. Juvenile homicide is, after all, a social and legal category, not a scientific construct, and there is no scientific basis for assuming that homicide by youths should be the product of a unique set of factors. Differences among violent youths will only obscure attempts to isolate factors that discriminate violent from nonviolent individuals. Future research should focus on identifying etiological factors associated with relatively homogeneous subgroups of violent youths.

4. Attempts to subgroup violent youths must adhere to standard procedures for proposing any diagnostic entity. There must be clear and reliable criteria for classifying subjects. The means by which youths are classified must be distinguished from findings used to support the validity of the classification. For example, the "nonempathic" murderers category proposed by Zenoff and Zients (1979) undoubtedly rings true for many forensic clinicians, yet the classification involves both the perpetrator-victim relationship, which is relatively objective, and a more inferential clinical opinion about the youth's personality development.

References

Adams KA: The child who murders: a review of theory and research. Criminal Justice and Behavior 1:51–61, 1974

Adelson L: The battering child. JAMA 222:159–161, 1972

Anthony EJ, Rizzo A: Adolescent girls who kill or try to kill their fathers, in The Child in His Family: The Impact of Disease and Death. Edited by Anthony EJ, Koupernik C. New York, Wiley Interscience, 1973

Bender L: Children and adolescents who have killed. Am J Psychiatry 116:510–513, 1959

Bender L, Curran FJ: Children and adolescents who kill. Journal of Criminal Psychopathology 1:196–322, 1940

Bender L, Keiser S, Schilder P: Studies in aggressiveness. Genetic Psychology Monographs 15:1937

Bernstein JI: Premeditated murder by an eight year old boy. International Journal of Offender Therapy and Comparative Criminology 22:47–56, 1978

Bunge M: Causality and Modern Science, 3rd edition, revised. New York, Dover Publications, 1979

Bureau of the Census: Preliminary Estimates of the Population of the United States, by Age, Sex, and Race: 1970 to 1981. Series P-25, no. 917. Washington, DC, U.S. Department of Commerce, 1982

Bureau of the Census: Estimates of the Population of the United States, by Age, Sex, and Race: 1980 to 1986. Series P-25, no. 1000. Washington, DC, U.S. Department of Commerce, 1987

Carek DJ, Watson AS: Treatment of a family involved in fratricide. Arch Gen Psychiatry 11:533–542, 1964

Corder BF, Ball BC, Haizlip TM, et al: Adolescent parricide: a comparison with other adolescent murder. Am J Psychiatry 133:957–961, 1976

Cormier B, Markus B: A longitudinal study of adolescent murderers. Bull Am Acad Psychiatry Law 8:240–260, 1980

Cormier B, Angliker C, Boyer R, et al: The psychodynamics of homicide committed in a specific relationship. Canadian Journal of Criminology and Corrections 13:1–8, 1971a

Cormier B, Angliker C, Boyer R, et al: The psychodynamics of homicide committed in a semi-specific relationship. Canadian Journal of Criminology and Corrections 14:335–344, 1971b

Cormier BM, Angliker CCJ, Gagne PW, et al: Adolescents who kill members of the family, in Family Violence: An International and Interdisciplinary Study. Edited by Eckclaar JM, Katz SN. Toronto, Butterworth, 1978, pp 466–478

Cornell D, Benedek E, Benedek D: Characteristics of adolescents charged with homicide: review of 72 cases. Behavioral Science and the Law 5:11–23, 1987a

Cornell D, Benedek E, Benedek D: Juvenile homicide: prior adjustment and a proposed typology. Am J Orthopsychiatry 57:383–393, 1987b

Cornell D, Miller C, Benedek E: MMPI profiles of adolescents charged with homicide. Behavioral Sciences and the Law 6:401–407, 1987c

Crowell DH, Evans IM, O'Donnell CR (eds): Childhood Aggression and Violence: Sources of Influence, Prevention, and Control. New York, Plenum, 1987

Duncan JW, Duncan GM: Murder in the family: a study of some homicidal adolescents. Am J Psychiatry 127:74–78, 1971

Easson WM, Steinhilber RM: Murderous aggression by children and adolescents. Arch Gen Psychiatry 4:1–9, 1961

Federal Bureau of Investigation: Uniform Crime Reports (1977–1986). Washington, DC, U.S. Government Printing Office, 1978–87

Gardiner M: The Deadly Innocents: Portraits of Children Who Kill. New Haven, Yale University Press, 1985

Greenberg HRO, Blank RH: Murder and self-destruction by a twelve-year-old boy. Adolescence 5:391–396, 1970

Grinker RR: What is the cause of violence? in Dynamics of Violence. Edited by Fawcett J. Chicago, American Medical Association, 1971

Haizlip T, Corder BF, Ball BC: The adolescent murderer, in The Aggressive Adolescent: Clinical Perspectives. Edited by Keith CR. New York, The Free Press, 1984

Hart HLA, Honoré T: Causation and the Law, 2nd edition. Oxford, Clarendon Press, 1985

Hays JR, Solway KS, Schreiner D: Intellectual characteristics of juvenile murderers versus status offenders. Psychol Rep 43:80–82, 1978

Hellsten P, Katila O: Murder and other homicide by children under 15 in Finland. Psychiatr Q (Suppl) 39:54–74, 1965

Kalogerakis MG: Homicide in adolescents: fantasy and deed, in Dynamics of Violence. Edited by Fawcett J. Chicago, American Medical Association, 1971

Keith CR (ed): The Aggressive Adolescent: Clinical Perspectives. New York, The Free Press, 1984

King CH: The ego and the integration of violence in homicidal youth. Am J Orthopsychiatry 45:134–145, 1975

Lewis DO: Vulnerabilities to Delinquency. New York, SP Medical and Scientific Books, 1981

Lewis DO, Shanok SS, Pincus JH: The neuropsychiatric status of violent male juvenile delinquents, in Vulnerabilities to Delinquency. Edited by Lewis DO. New York, SP Medical and Scientific Books, 1981

Lewis DO, Shanok SS, Grant M, et al: Homicidally aggressive young children: neuropsychiatric and experiential correlates. Am J Psychiatry 140:148–153, 1983

Lewis DO, Moy E, Jackson LD, et al: Biopsychosocial characteristics of children who later murder: a prospective study. Am J Psychiatry 142:1161–1167, 1985

Lochman JE: Psychological characteristics and assessment of aggressive adolescents, in The Aggressive Adolescent: Clinical Perspectives. Edited by Keith CR. New York, The Free Press, 1984

Mack J, Scherl D, Macht L: Children who kill their mothers, in The Child in His Family: The Impact of Disease and Death. Edited by Anthony EJ, Koupernik C. New York, Wiley Interscience, 1973

Malmquist CP: Premonitory signs of homicidal aggression in juveniles. Am J Psychiatry 128:93–97, 1971

McCarthy J: Narcissism and the self in homicidal adolescents. Am J Psychoanal 38:19–29, 1978

Medlicott RW: Paranoia of the exalted type in a setting of *folie à deux:* a study of two adolescent homicides. Br J Med Psychol 28:205–223, 1955

Menninger K, Mayman M: Episodic dyscontrol: a third order of stress adaptation. Bull Menninger Clin 20:153–165, 1956

Michaels JJ: Enuresis in murderous aggressive children and adolescents. Arch Gen Psychiatry 5:94–97, 1961

Miller D, Looney J: The prediction of adolescent homicide: episodic dyscontrol and dehumanization. Am J Psychoanal 34:187–198, 1974

Mohr JW, McKnight CK: Violence as a function of age and relationship with special reference to matricide. Can Psychiatr Assoc 16:29–32, 1971

Mones P: The relationship between child abuse and parricide, in Unhapppy Families: Clinical and Research Perspectives on Family Violence. Edited by Newberg EH, Bourne R. Littleton, MA, PSG Publishing, 1985

Morris G: The Kids Next Door: Sons and Daughters Who Kill Their Parents. New York, William Morrow, 1985

Paluszny M, McNabb M: Therapy of a six-year-old who committed fratricide. J Am Acad Child Psychiatry 14: 319–336, 1975

Patterson RM: Psychiatric study of juveniles involved in homicide. Am J Orthopsychiatry 13:125–130, 1943

Petti TA, Davidman L: Homicidal school-age children: cognitive style and demographic features. Child Psychiatry Hum Dev 12:82–89, 1981

Pfeffer CR: Psychiatric hospital treatment of assaultive homicidal children. Am J Psychother 34:197–207, 1980

Pope HG, Jonas JM, Hudson JI, et al: An empirical study of psychosis in borderline personality disorder. Am J Psychiatry 142:1285–1290, 1985

Post S: Adolescent parricide in abusive families. Child Welfare 61(7):445–455, 1982

Reinhardt JM: Nothing Left But . . . Murder. Lincoln, NE, Johnsen Publishing, 1970

Rogers R: Conducting Insanity Evaluations. New York, Van Nostrand Reinhold, 1986

Rosner R, Weiderlight M, Rosner MB, et al: Adolescents accused of murder and manslaughter: a five year descriptive study. Bull Am Acad Psychiatry Law 7:342–351, 1978

Rowley JC, Ewing CP, Singer SI: Juvenile homicide: the need for an interdisciplinary approach. Behavioral Sciences and the Law 5:1–10, 1987

Russell DH: A study of juvenile murderers. Journal of Offender Therapy 9:55–86, 1965

Russell DH: Juvenile murderers. International Journal of Offender Therapy and Comparative Criminology 18: 235–239, 1973

Russell DH: Ingredients of juvenile murder. International Journal of Offender Therapy and Comparative Criminology 23:65–72, 1979

Sadoff RL: Clinical observation on parricide. Psychiatr Q 45:65–69, 1971

Sargent D: Children who kill—a family conspiracy? Social Work 7:35–42, 1962

Sargent D: The lethal situation: transmission of urge to kill from patient to child, in Dynamics of Violence. Edited by Fawcett J. Chicago, American Medical Association, 1971

Satten J, Menninger K, Rosen I, et al: Murder without apparent motive: a study in personality disorganization. Am J Psychiatry 117:18–53, 1960

Schacter DL: Amnesia and crime: how much do we really know? Am Psychol 41:286–295, 1986

Scherl DJ, Mack JE: A study of adolescent matricide. J Am Acad Child Psychiatry 5:559–593, 1966

Schmideberg M: Juvenile murderers. International Journal of Offender Therapy and Comparative Criminology 17:240–245, 1973

Sendi, IB, Blomgren PG: A comparative study of predictive criteria in the predisposition of homicidal adolescents. Am J Psychiatry 132:423–428, 1975

Smith S: The adolescent murderer: a psychodynamic interpretation. Arch Gen Psychiatry 13:310–319, 1965

Solway KS, Richardson L, Hays JR, et al: Adolescent murderers: literature review and preliminary research findings, in Violence and the Violent Individual. Edited by Hays JR, Roberts TK, Solway KS. New York, SP Medical and Scientific Books, 1981

Sorrells JM: Kids who kill. Crime and Delinquency 23: 312–320, 1977

Sorrells JM: What can be done about juvenile homicide? Crime and Delinquency 26:152–161, 1980

Stearns A: Murder by adolescents with obscure motivation. Am J Psychiatry 114:303–305, 1957

Tanay E: Adolescents who kill parents—reactive parricide. Aust N Z J Psychiatry 7:263–277, 1973

Tanay E: Reactive parricide. Journal of Forensic Sciences 21:76–82, 1976

Thornton WE, Pray BJ: The portrait of a murderer. Dis Nerv Syst 36:176–178, 1975

Tooley K: The small assassins: clinical notes on a subgroup of murderous children. J Am Acad Child Psychiatry 14:306–336, 1975

Tracy PE, Wolfgang ME, Figlio RM: Delinquency in Two Birth Cohorts. Washington, DC, U.S. Department of Justice, 1985

Tucker LS, Cornwall TP: Mother-son *folie à deux:* a case of attempted patricide. Am J Psychiatry 134:1146–1147, 1977

Walshe-Brennan KS: An analysis of homicide by young persons in England and Wales. Acta Psychiatr Scand 54:92–98, 1976

Walshe-Brennan KS: A socio-psychological investigation of young murderers. British Journal of Criminology 17(1):53–63, 1977

Wittman P, Astrachan M: Psychological investigation of a homicidal youth. J Clin Psychol 5:88–93, 1949

Wolfgang ME: Patterns in Criminal Homicide. Philadelphia, University of Pennsylvania Press, 1958

Wolfgang ME, Figlio RM, Sellin T: Delinquency in a Birth Cohort. Chicago, University of Chicago Press, 1972

Woods SM: Adolescent violence and homicide: ego disruption and the 6 and 14 dysrhythmia. Arch Gen Psychiatry 5:528–534, 1961

Yates A, Beutler LE, Crago M: Characteristics of young, violent offenders. Journal of Psychiatry and Law 137–149, 1984

Zenoff EH, Zients AB: Juvenile murderers: should the punishment fit the crime? Int J Law Psychiatry 2:533–553, 1979

Chapter 2

Clinical Presentations of Homicidal Adolescents

ELISSA P. BENEDEK, M.D.
DEWEY G. CORNELL, Ph.D.

Chapter 2

Clinical Presentations of Homicidal Adolescents

Societal response to juvenile violence is a challenge for the psychiatrist, psychologist, sociologist, or attorney, because at best it is ambivalent. Public debate ranges between extreme responses such as psychiatric treatment or incarceration, rehabilitation or capital punishment. Traditionally, responsibility for society's response to adolescent homicide has been left to the law and the criminal justice system. However, despite the valiant efforts of law enforcement, judicial, and penal personnel, homicide is one of the five leading causes of death for all persons in the United States who are 1 to 17 years of age, and most homicides are committed by youths or young adults. Although juveniles who kill represent a small fraction of homicide perpetrators, they too present a major challenge to courts and clinicians. We know very little about youngsters who kill. We know less about why they kill and even less about whether an individual adolescent will behave violently in the future.

Adolescent Homicides in Michigan

The youngsters described in this chapter are drawn from a sample of adolescents charged with homicide whom we have studied in the state of Michigan. We use the term *adolescent* to refer to youths as old as 18 and *homicide* to include first or second degree murder, but not deaths attributable to accident or self-defense. We recognize that this sample is not necessarily representative of all adolescents who commit homicide. As detailed in Chapter 3, our sample of 72 youths consisted of only a small percentage of all the youths arrested for homicide in Michigan during the time period (1977–1985) of our study. In addition, our sample was limited to cases referred by the courts to the Michigan Center for Forensic Psychiatry for psychiatric evaluation.

Nevertheless, the 72 youths we studied were quite diverse in the background and circumstances of their offenses, and especially in their clinical presentations. In this chapter we demonstrate the heterogeneity and complexity of adolescent homicide by reviewing a series of contrasting cases. Our clinical experiences led us to conclude that simple comparisons between these youths and other delinquent groups would be of limited value and not lead to useful generalizations. As a result, we felt it essential to classify adolescent murderers into subgroups. In Chapter 3 we present research on a three-group typology of adolescent murderers, which we feel capture some, but not all, of the important clinical distinctions necessary to understand the nature of adolescent homicide.

We classified youths into one of three general categories based on their mental state and the circumstances of the offense: 1) youths who were psychotic at the time of the offense; 2) youths who committed homicide in association with another crime (for example, robbery or rape); and 3) youths who committed homicide in association with an interpersonal conflict with the victim. (Coding criteria and examples are available from Cornell.) Information describing the circumstances of the offense and the defendant's behavior at this time was used to classify each case. This information came from detailed police reports including review of the crime scene, accounts of witnesses, statements made by defendants at the time of arrest, and the defendant's account of the offense during a forensic evaluation conducted by experienced forensic clinicians.

The Question of Psychosis

The question of psychosis is critical to a forensic evaluation because the presence of psychotic symptoms can support an insanity defense. In this project, defendants were classified as psychotic at the time of the offense if they met DSM-III criteria (American Psychiatric Association 1980) for psychosis. The psychosis could be due to drug intoxication, schizophrenia, major affective disorder, or any other psychiatric disorder. For the youths in this group who were psychotic, the most common and clear-cut indications of psychosis were hallucinations and delusions. Less often, the psychosis was manifested by grossly bizarre behavior at the time of a crime, for example, tearing off one's clothing, drinking one's urine, or painting a victim's nipples and vagina after a murder.

One difficult problem in diagnosis reported by clinicians occurred when a defendant claimed psychotic symptoms but appeared to be malingering. In a general forensic psychiatric population, approximately 7–10 percent of the defendants could be diagnosed as malingering their psychotic symptoms, according to evaluations conducted by experienced forensic examiners (Cornell and Hawk, in press). It is reasonable to assume that a similar proportion of adolescent homicide defendants might attempt to malinger, too, whether out of fear, in hopes of avoiding trial, or in an attempt to manipulate the outcome of a clinical evaluation.

In difficult cases, it was possible to make an assessment of malingering by reviewing 1) independent reports of bizarre behavior by the defendant at the time of the offense as compared to the defendant's own self-report; 2) independent reports of history of psychosis or severe psychiatric disorder; 3) the quality of symptoms presented by the defendant (that is, whether the symptoms were obviously feigned, such as "smoke coming out of my fingers and ears"); 4) the convincing and unwavering nature of the defendant's symptoms over time, especially over the course of inpatient observation; and 5) evaluation by

41

an experienced clinician. We did not consider defendants psychotic if they made vague statements such as "I was out of my head" or "I must have been crazy," or "The Devil made me do it."

The small number of youngsters who feigned psychotic symptoms seemed to do so early in the forensic evaluation process. These youngsters also were more likely to have had contact with either the juvenile justice system or the mental health system in the past. This contact afforded them an opportunity to observe severely disturbed youngsters and mimic symptoms that others had exhibited. In such cases these youngsters often admitted to feigned symptoms when confronted by an experienced examiner. In other cases, the youngsters recanted their symptoms when the examiner talked with them about their fears and fantasies of forensic evaluations, the trial process, hospitalization, or the juvenile justice system.

In rare cases, although a more experienced forensic examiner might believe that a youngster was feigning mental illness, the court can be convinced by an independent examiner (with less forensic experience) that the illness was genuine. Because of the importance of assessing malingering in forensic evaluations, we begin with a case of feigned mental illness.

A Case of Feigned Mental Illness

Sampson, a 16-year-old, single white male was charged with first degree murder in the death of his 13-year-old sister. The defendant's sister was found by her father at home lying on the living room floor. She had been stabbed by a knife and struck repeatedly on the head with a metal pipe. The defendant was also found lying on the floor, with minor injuries.

Initially, Sampson told police that he and his sister had been attacked by two intruders. Later, he identified them as Mike and Jimmy, two teenagers who had teased him at school in the past. However, upon further questioning, there were inconsistencies in Sampson's account, and officers began to suspect that he might have been the assailant.

Forensic evaluation. Sampson was referred for outpatient evaluation of competency to stand trial and criminal responsibility (insanity). At this time, the defendant reported visual and auditory hallucinations of several persons who came to visit him in his jail cell. Primary among them was "Evil Guy," a demonlike figure who told him to "do bad things," such as kill his mother. He maintained that he had been troubled by the specter of the Evil Guy for some time preceding the offense but had not told anyone, including his therapist. He told the examiner that he had given the police a false statement immediately after the offense because he was frightened of them and actually did not remember what transpired.

Sampson claimed minimal understanding of his legal situation and began to talk in a childlike manner. For example, when asked what might occur should he be convicted of the offense, he stated, "I might go away," but only "until my ma came and got me."

The defendant was adjudicated incompetent to stand trial and admitted to the Forensic Center. Eventually, he gave an account of the offense. This included an account of a typical day at school, his return home, and watching television with his sister. He reported that suddenly, without explanation, the Evil Guy made him start hitting and stabbing his sister until she was dead.

Sampson described the Evil Guy in great detail. He stated that he could "make people kill and destroy things and make you not love and take away the people you love." He had seen Evil Guy for three years before the homicide, but had told no one.

In clinical interviews Sampson complained about being disturbed by Evil Guy, but ward staff observed no unusual behavior or signs of distraction by internal stimuli. He interacted well with other patients and took part in ward activities. No medication was prescribed because he never evidenced psychotic symptoms beyond his self-reported hallucinations.

Sampson had received psychological testing prior to the offense. On the Wechsler Intelligence Scale for Children, Revised (WISC-R), he obtained a full scale IQ of 118, placing him in the high average range of intellectual functioning. On the Minnesota Multiphasic Personality Inventory (MMPI), his clinical scores were all within the average range.

During Sampson's hospitalization at the Forensic Center, he was given additional testing. This time his performance reflected clear tendencies to exaggerate or malinger symptoms of mental illness. He refused to answer many WISC-R questions that he answered easily before and undoubtedly were above his current level of day-to-day functioning. He took the MMPI on three occasions over a nine-month period, each time producing an invalid profile with extreme elevations on almost all clinical scales.

History.   Sampson was one of two adopted children. He denied any problems or difficulties in his family, but in fact had a history of serious alcohol and drug abuse (marijuana and amphetamines), lying, and stealing in the home. He had previously beaten his sister. He was truant and made poor grades in school. A year prior to the offense, his parents took him for psychotherapy. His therapist reported, "At no time did Sampson exhibit any signs of a thought disorder or serious mental illness." The defendant claimed that he had tried to tell his therapist about Evil Guy, but that the therapist did not want to hear about it and kept insisting on talking about school work.

Forensic outcome.   Based on his unusual and highly inconsistent clinical presentation, and extensive evaluation, clinicians at the Forensic Center concluded that Sampson was malingering and did not meet criteria for legal insanity. In contrast, an independent examiner, who interviewed the defendant but failed to review his clinical records or interview his parents, concluded that he was insane. The jury found the defendant not guilty by reason of insanity. When interviewed, a juror stated, "The murder was so bizarre he had to be crazy."

As a result of his acquittal, the defendant was required to undergo an evaluation to determine whether he met criteria for civil commitment as mentally ill and dangerous to himself or others. At this evaluation, Sampson presented no symptoms of mental illness. He denied that he experienced any symptoms or needed treatment. A court hearing found him not committable and he was released to the community.

A Case of Genuine Psychosis

Seventeen-year-old Allen was charged with murder in the stabbing death of a 16-year-old male peer. The victim was found lying in a drainage ditch near his home. At the time of his arrest, the defendant told police that he was "under lots of pressure" from the "radio and TV giving me ideas . . . that I had to kill . . . like Baretta."

Forensic evaluation.   Allen acknowledged the killing, stating that "destiny led me," and that "Jesus died on the cross for me so I wouldn't have to die, but I could kill somebody else so we both could die." His account of his behavior was disorganized and replete with confused and delusional thinking. At one point he announced, "I am Jesus Christ Superstar, Bob Seger, José Wales." He reported that music on the radio was directed specifically to him and referred to him as "the Lord." He also heard "a violent voice" that "told me to kill."

An extensive neurological workup including neurological exam, x-rays, and EEG revealed no signs of organic difficulties. Psychological testing supported the diagnosis of paranoid schizophrenia.

Initially, Allen was found incompetent to stand trial and was committed for hospital treatment. After several months of treatment with psychotropic medication and supportive therapy, he showed a very modest degree of improvement and was judged to be marginally competent to return to court.

History. Allen was the oldest of four male siblings. His mother had been hospitalized numerous times for psychiatric illness, and his father had cared for the children during his mother's absence. There was an extensive history of schizophrenia and schizophrenic symptoms on his maternal side. Allen had no history of involvement with juvenile authorities. He was an average student and was described as seclusive, but well-behaved, in school.

Allen had a three-year history of serious mental disorder. He described an abrupt and dramatic onset of symptomatology including religious delusions, visual hallucinations, and other symptoms of serious thought disorder. He was hospitalized three times in his local community prior to his offense. The most recent hospitalization had occurred when he tried to drown his two younger brothers, ages 12 and 6.

During his previous psychiatric hospitalizations Allen had described extensive delusions of reference and was assaultive toward staff. He also attempted to provoke other patients to assault him. After each discharge he discontinued his psychotropic medication and underwent a gradual decline that resulted in rehospitalization.

Forensic outcome. The forensic examiner testified that Allen suffered from a mental disorder that met criteria for legal insanity. He was found not guilty by reason of insanity after a bench trial and was committed to the Forensic Center for evaluation of his need for civil commitment. He was judged in need of involuntary treatment and has remained in an inpatient treatment program for four years. Treatment has consisted of a complete therapeutic program including inpatient hospitalization, supportive psychotherapy, ancillary therapy (such as school, occupational therapy, and recreational therapy), neuroleptic medications, and lithium. Allen has remained refractory to treatment and is intermittently acutely psychotic. His family has abandoned him and is not part of the treatment program.

A Second Psychotic Case

Fifteen-year-old Bob was charged with the murder of his mother. One afternoon his father returned home from work to discover his wife stabbed to death. Bob was found by his father hiding in the basement, reading the Bible, and chanting, "Kill the Devil."

Forensic evaluation. Upon evaluation after the offense, Bob continued to profess a strong belief in witchcraft. He claimed that he had listened to rock music the day of the crime and that he had heard special messages on his phonograph that were directed to him and suggested that he kill his mother. Bob had little idea of the seriousness of the charges against him and believed he would be saved by Satan. The forensic examiner recommended that he not be waived to adult court and that he be found incompetent to stand trial.

History. Bob had been known to argue regularly with his abusive mother. He ran away from home two times after violent quarrels and on one occasion was temporarily housed in a facility for serious offenders. On at least one occasion, Bob and his mother had a physical altercation and had to be separated by the boy's father.

For two months prior to the homicide, Bob had become progressively more withdrawn, violent, and apathetic. He remained secluded in his room listening to music. Although his prior friendships had been few, he refused to speak to any of his friends. His school attendance was sporadic. He paced through the night and began to talk about "witchcraft" and "demonic possession." He refused to eat, claiming that his mother was poisoning his food.

Forensic outcome. Bob was committed to a state adolescent inpatient facility as incompetent to stand trial. He was reported to be responding well to a program of inpatient hospitalization, psychotherapy, neuroleptic medications, and milieu therapy. Although responding to treatment, he remains hospitalized because his psychotic episode has been followed by a serious depression and he is now considered a suicide risk.

Homicide Committed During Another Crime

The next group of youngsters are those who committed a homicide in the course of another criminally motivated act such as robbery, burglary, or rape. Other investigators have noted a similar subgroup (Solway et al. 1981; Zenoff and Zients 1979).

Rosenaur (1983) reports that between 1976 and 1979, only 17 percent of homicides in the United States were committed during the course of another crime such as robbery or burglary. In our sample, however, 52 percent of the youngsters committed their homicide in the course of another crime (see Chapter 3). This homicide was most often secondary to the other crime and often unplanned. For example, the victim might awaken during a burglary, scream, and as a result of this behavior be killed. This group of murderers also included a contract murderer—that is, a murder that was paid for by an organized crime organization. Most typically the victims in this group were strangers, but a number of crime homicide victims also included neighbors and acquaintances. In one case, a defendant did murder a family member in order to assume control of the family business and collect the fire insurance from a burned building.

Homicide Associated with Rape and Robbery

Charlie was a 16-year-old charged with first degree murder, criminal sexual conduct, and unarmed robbery involving an elderly woman. The woman's partially nude body was found in her home. She had been severely beaten, with a fractured skull and wounds to her arms, legs, and vaginal area.

Forensic evaluation.   During the forensic evaluation, the defendant stated bluntly, "I did it. I hit her with a stick." Detailed questioning revealed that on the day of the murder the defendant spent the afternoon visiting with friends, drinking beer, and smoking pot. He told the examiner, "I remember I had a buzz on. A pretty strong buzz." After leaving his friend's home, he walked down the street and decided to look in the window of the victim's house. He reported, "I was looking in her front windows thinking should I go in or what. I was thinking about having sex or something. I thought I might have sex with her if I went in." Charlie related, "I went in and said, 'Are you going to give me what I want?' And she said, 'No, get out of my house.' And then I took a stick and I hit her."

The defendant presented no indications of mental illness past or present. Below-average intelligence was confirmed by intelligence testing.

History.   Charlie's parents separated when he was five, and he grew up in his mother's custody. He reported a good relationship with his mother, but recalled that his father had been physically abusive of his mother on many occasions. Charlie had been a poor student in school and dropped out after completing the seventh grade. He reported that he began experimenting with alcohol in the fourth grade and that his drinking increased gradually over the years to include weekend binges and moderate drinking every evening.

Charlie had several prior charges of criminal sexual conduct and unarmed robbery that had been dismissed. He had spent several months in a training school for joyriding.

Forensic outcome.   The forensic examiner recommended that the defendant be waived to adult court and that he be found competent and criminally responsible. Charlie was waived to adult court and agreed to a plea bargain for second degree murder. Currently he is in prison.

Homicide Associated with Robbery

Sixteen-year-old Donald and his friend, Ernie, were charged with murder in the death of a male vagrant.

Forensic evaluation. Donald admitted that he and Ernie made a habit of robbing street beggars when they needed extra cash. One of the street people resisted and Donald hit the old man over the head with a brick, killing him. He and his companion pocketed the money and ran. Donald stated that he did not intend to kill the old man, but when the "tramp" called them names and spit on them, it made him "so mad" that he had to "get even."

Forensic outcome. Donald and his friend were not waived from juvenile court into adult court. They were sentenced in the juvenile court, served one year in a training school, and returned to the community.

A Female Charged with Homicide

Sixteen-year-old Eve was charged with first degree murder, conspiracy to murder, kidnapping, and armed robbery involving a 50-year-old man. The victim was known as Mr. Quick, a wealthy divorcee who had a reputation in the community for cruising through town and picking up adolescent females for sexual favors. Initially, the police received a call from Mr. Quick, who reported being kidnapped and beaten by three women. He was admitted to a local hospital, but he died of complications associated with a broken collarbone and internal injuries.

Forensic evaluation. Eve acknowledged her participation in the murder, but claimed that she had been "manipulated" by her two older female friends, one of whom had a prison record. According to Eve, her friends convinced her to let Mr. Quick pick her up and take her back to his house. The two friends joined her at the house and attempted to seduce Mr. Quick. Apparently, Mr. Quick became suspicious and attempted to use the phone, but the women intervened and struck him with a hammer and a chain. They forced him into the trunk of his automobile and drove to a nearby city. Here they again beat Mr. Quick and then dumped him in an alley. Subsequently, they found a purchaser for the car and used the money to obtain cocaine and transportation home.

In the next few days, the women began a crime spree that included robbing a blind woman and her disabled husband. They were apprehended by police while attempting to sell the couple's automobile.

History. Eve was a middle child in a sibship of four. Her mother was described as a strict woman who repeatedly told her "not to hang around with people who are no good." However, her mother was responsible for her early release from juvenile detention on both occasions and vouched for her continuing good behavior. Her father was disabled, and she reported that she got along well with him "because he didn't give me no trouble."

Eve had eight previous arrests, including at least two violent offenses that resulted in placement in a juvenile detention center. On one occasion, she had beaten an older woman and stolen her money. On another, she had robbed a blind man. Eve dropped out of school during the tenth grade. Her substance abuse history included use of alcohol, marijuana, PCP, and cocaine.

Forensic outcome. Eve was recommended for waiver to adult court. She was convicted of all charges and sentenced to prison at the women's correctional facility.

Conflict-Related Homicides

In our third group, the homicide was related to an ongoing interpersonal conflict with the victim. The defendant generally was involved in a prolonged argument or dispute, although the homicide was not necessarily carried out during an argument and could have been planned over a period of time. Frequently the perpetrator might have acted in anticipation of a renewal of the ongoing conflict. A typical situation involved an adolescent male who, after years of conflict with parental authority, planned and carried out an ambush of his abusive father.

These defendants almost always had some history of prior conflict with the victim. In rare cases, the relationship was brief. For example, in one case, an adolescent murdered an acquaintance after a brief homosexual encounter. In these situations, there was also a clear absence of psychosis and an absence of another criminal act such as robbery or rape. In an occasional case, the defendant stole from the victim after the homicide or committed an arson. For example, one young perpetrator murdered his father, stole his father's money, and then set his father's house on fire in an attempt to conceal the homicide. This boy tried to disguise what happened by writing a note stating that he was being kidnapped and then left the state.

Murder of an Abusive Father

Fred was a 17-year-old boy charged with first degree murder in the death of his father. Fred shot his father in the living room and then called police to report what happened. After the police arrived, they found Fred sobbing uncontrollably and all that they were able to understand was the boy saying, "I shot my daddy."

Forensic evaluation. Fred described a long history of abuse of himself and his siblings by his father. The homicide occurred during another violent episode in which father was beating the defendant's sister. Fred reported that, after his father stopped momentarily to go to the bathroom, he retrieved his father's rifle from the bedroom. When father came out of the bedroom, Fred shot him without warning.

History. There was an extensive history of physical abuse of all family members by the father. The account given by Fred, and corroborated by family members and neighbors, depicted the father as an alcoholic who was extremely brutal and tyrannical. The father's abuse of Fred's mother had precipitated her suicide when Fred was 13. The defendant vividly recalled the argument between his father and mother prior to the suicide. His distraught mother locked herself in her bedroom and threatened to shoot herself. Over the next few hours, the father used Fred to relay messages to her. During this time Fred heard the gunshot as his mother shot herself.

Fred reported that his father beat his second wife, too. He not only whipped his children, he made the older ones administer "punishment" to the younger ones. Thus Fred had not only been the recipient of physical abuse, on some occasions he had been made to administer his father's abuse to his younger siblings as well.

Fred did not have a previous psychiatric or criminal history. Despite his obviously traumatic experiences, he was never referred for counseling. He made above-average grades in school and had graduated from high school one year early.

Forensic outcome. Fred raised an insanity defense at his bench trial. Testifying psychiatric experts differed as to whether he was legally insane at the time of the crime, but the judge acquitted him as insane. He underwent an inpatient evaluation and was found to have no current symptoms that would justify involuntary civil commitment. He was discharged with a recommendation for outpatient treatment.

Murder of a Peer

Gary was a 15-year-old boy charged with first degree murder in the death of a 14-year-old peer, Betsy. The girl was found stabbed to death in her home one day after school. Physical evidence at the scene implicated the boy as a suspect, and upon questioning three days later, he confessed to the crime.

Forensic evaluation. Gary was initially very reticent and required multiple interviews before rapport was established. Eventually, he was willing to describe the offense. He related that he had been very angry with Betsy for several weeks, and on the day of the offense went to her house after school to "straighten things out." However, he lost his temper and attacked her with a kitchen knife. Afterwards, he went home and tried to pretend that nothing had happened. There was considerable mystery around Gary's motives for the offense, although a complicated picture slowly emerged. Initially, Gary offered no motive, but later he reported that he killed Betsy because she teased him at school. Gary complained that many students made fun of him because of his appearance, especially his facial acne. Betsy had initiated calling him "crater-face," a term that others took up as well.

However, the examiner was not satisfied that being teased was a sufficient motive for the homicide and questioned Gary further. In fact, Gary knew Betsy very well because their parents were divorced and his mother had dated Betsy's father. Gary found that his mother was spending more and more time with Betsy's father, and this meant that he also had to spend time with Betsy. There were hints that Gary may have had a "crush" on Betsy, but he denied it, and in any event, Betsy made it clear that she wanted nothing to do with him. She constantly made fun of him. Eventually, he acknowledged that one of her final remarks to him before he attacked her was to jeer at him that he would never have a girlfriend.

In the weeks prior to the homicide, Gary had become depressed over his mother's increasing involvement with Betsy's father. He was angry that he had to spend time with Betsy, but he was also clearly jealous that his mother spent so much time with Betsy's father. Gary's mother described him as becoming depressed and withdrawn, but she was unaware of the reason for his change in mood. She knew that he disliked Betsy and complained about her teasing him, but had no idea of the depth of his feeling. It was noteworthy that the weekend prior to the homicide, Gary had been sick with the flu. He complained that his mother went out with Betsy's father anyway, leaving him home alone.

Gary eventually acknowledged that he had contemplated killing Betsy for several weeks prior to the homicide. He reported that the idea had come to him in a dream. This led to extensive investigation of his mental state and review of any possible psychotic symptoms, as well as examination for major depression. After repeated interviews, including the Kiddie Schedule for Affective Disorders and Schizophrenia (SADS) and a battery of psychological tests, there was no evidence of psychotic thinking or experiences. Gary appeared to be a deeply conflicted, depressed, and ruminative youth who nevertheless had intact reality testing. His level of depression was noteworthy, but did not meet criteria for a major depressive episode either before or after the offense.

Several factors seem to have motivated Gary in his homicidal behavior. He was angry and resentful of Betsy because she teased and humiliated him in front of his peers. This hurt was magnified by his feelings of attraction for her and her emphatic rejection of him. Ordinarily, Gary might simply have avoided Betsy and forgotten about her, but the fact that their parents were dating brought him into continual contact with her. The prospect that their parents might marry meant that Betsy would become his stepsister, trapping him with the person he hated for rejecting him and teasing him.

A further complication was that Gary's anger with Betsy may have represented an expression of his resentment and jealousy over his mother dating her father. He was opposed to the marriage and experienced it as a rejection that his mother seemed to turn from him to another. The possibility of unconscious oedipal conflicts, heightened by the incestuous quality of his feelings for a prospective sister, would deserve exploration in the course of long-term psychotherapy.

History.   Gary's parents had divorced when he was in grade school. He maintained contact with both parents, and the two of them were on good terms. There was no history of physical or sexual abuse in the family. Gary had never been in trouble with juvenile authorities and was viewed as a quiet, well-behaved youngster. There was no indication of alcohol or substance abuse. He had a small group of male friends but had not dated girls. His grades had been average throughout his school years, but prior to the offense they had dropped so much that he was in danger of failing several classes.

Forensic outcome. Despite extensive investigation, the forensic examiner could find no basis for concluding that Gary suffered from a mental illness fitting statutory criteria for insanity. He was tried in adult court, convicted of second degree murder, and sentenced to prison.

Conclusion

The purpose of our initial research was to study clinical features of adolescent homicide. We believe that the discrepant characterizations of these youths reported in the literature were in part the product of small sample sizes and a failure to recognize important clinical distinctions among adolescent subgroups. This larger sample enabled us to differentiate three distinct clinical groups. We believe that relatively straightforward clinical distinctions such as these can provide a basis for progress in future research on the etiology, assessment, and treatment of severely violent youths.

References

American Psychiatric Association: Diagnostic and Statistical Manual of Mental Disorders, Third edition. Washington, DC, American Psychiatric Association, 1980

Cornell DG, Hawk GL: Clinical presentation of malingerers: cases diagnosed by experienced forensic examiners. Law and Human Behavior (in press)

Solway KS, Richardson L, Hays JR, et al: Adolescent murderers: literature review and preliminary research findings, in Violence and the Violent Individual. Edited by Hays JR, Roberts TK, Solway KS. New York, SP Medical and Scientific Books, 1981

U.S. Department of Justice: Report to the Nation on Crime and Justice: The Data. Washington, DC, U.S. Department of Justice, Bureau of Juvenile Statistics, 1983

Zenoff EH, Zients AB: Juvenile murderers: should the punishment fit the crime? International Journal of Law and Psychiatry 2:533–553, 1979

Chapter 3

A Typology of Juvenile Homicide Offenders

DEWEY G. CORNELL, Ph.D.
ELISSA P. BENEDEK, M.D.
DAVID M. BENEDEK

Chapter 3

A Typology of Juvenile Homicide Offenders

As reviewed in Chapter 1, the literature amply documents the clinical diversity of adolescents who commit homicide, as well as the equal diversity in theories and viewpoints about the etiology of their homicidal behavior. A major contention of this chapter is that the lack of cumulative progress in research on juvenile homicide is attributable to a basic problem in conceptualization and research design: Violent behavior is too global a construct to study through simple comparisons of violent and nonviolent subjects. Violent individuals are a heterogeneous group that cannot be distinguished reliably and systematically from nonviolent individuals. Instead, the concept of violent behavior must be refined to incorporate multiple subgroups that are themselves distinguishable from one another, and in this way are individually distinguishable from nonviolent groups.

As Edwin Megargee (1970) observed nearly 20 years ago:

> Instead of attempting to predict "violence" as if it was a unitary, homogeneous mode of behavior, efforts should be directed at differentiating meaningful subtypes or syndromes of violent individuals and then determining the diagnostic signs in the clinical data that will enable us to identify individuals of each type. (p. 146)

Information contained in this chapter is based in part on previous articles published in the *American Journal of Orthopsychiatry* (57:383–393, 1987) and in *Behavioral Sciences and the Law* (5:11–23, 1987).

For example, in reviewing research with the Minnesota Multiphasic Personality Inventory (MMPI), Megargee (1970) observed that numerous studies failed to find differences between violent and nonviolent comparison groups, including both criminal and noncriminal populations. However, MMPI research that first distinguished among meaningful subtypes of violent individuals was much more successful (Megargee 1970).

Although many authorities would agree that individuals are violent for different reasons, the full implications of this view have not been adequately appreciated, nor have they been reflected in most of the research literature. Researchers continue to make global contrasts of violent and nonviolent comparison groups, in the dim hope that there will be sufficient homogeneity among violent individuals to distinguish them from nonviolent controls (Monahan 1981; Olweus 1980; Roth 1985).

The most compelling way to establish the *necessity* of a differentiated approach to juvenile homicide, and to human violent behavior in general, is to demonstrate clear and pervasive differences *within* a group of severely violent individuals. To be maximally useful and valid, *differences among violent youths should be evident not only in the circumstances of the violent behavior but in factors external to the violence as well.* Such factors might include the youth's family and developmental background, personality, and prior adjustment.

A Typology of Adolescents Who Commit Homicide

In our research, we attempted a more sophisticated approach to the study of juvenile violence by devising a typology that would capture some of the major distinctions among juvenile homicide offenders suggested in the literature. In our view, many previous conceptions of juvenile homicide seem to cluster into three main categories.

One long-standing conception in the literature is that the

62

juvenile murderer is psychotic or at least has severe ego weaknesses that result in brief, psychotic episodes (Bender 1959; Satten et al. 1960; Sendi and Blomgren 1975). Clearly, it seems important to distinguish juveniles suffering from severe mental illness (that is, psychosis) from others who commit homicide.

A second view is that these adolescents are products of severely disturbed and chaotic families and act in response to intense interpersonal and/or intrapsychic conflict (Adams 1974; Corder et al. 1976; McCarthy 1977). Special attention has focused on adolescents who appear to act out covert family pressures to murder an abusive parent or stepparent (Cormier et al. 1978; Duncan and Duncan 1971; Sargent 1962).

Relatively less attention has been given to homicides committed in the course of some other criminal activity such as robbery or rape, despite the broad literature on aggressive delinquents (Keith 1984; Wolfgang et al. 1972). The law recognizes the importance of this distinction in many jurisdictions that distinguish so-called "felony murders" from other forms of murder. These types of cases may be less likely to come to the attention of clinicians drawing their samples from psychiatric settings or independent practice. However, Zenoff and Zients (1979) do refer to "nonempathic" murderers who kill in the course of other criminal activity or without apparent motivating conflict with the victim. Solway and colleagues (1981) note a similar distinction.

It would seem most useful for both clinical and legal purposes if a typology were based on circumstances surrounding the offense and characteristics of the adolescent at this time. Although classification could not in itself determine clinical opinion on forensic questions such as competency to stand trial or legal insanity, clinicians would have available an empirically based source of information about juvenile homicide to assist in the evaluation process. This would provide a potential framework for conceptualizing the case and offer a way to clarify the various clinical presentations of juveniles charged with homicide. Classification based on circumstances of the offense would have potential relevance to legal decision making because it is linked directly to the illegal act. Validation of the typology would rest on factors external to the offense, such as the adolescent's developmental background or prior adjustment.

The present study investigated a typology that attempted to encompass some of the major group distinctions hypothesized in the literature, but that was restricted to classification criteria drawn from the circumstances of the offense. The classification scheme emphasized relatively staightforward distinctions among the following three groups: 1) *Psychotic* group, adolescents with clear psychotic symptoms (delusions, hallucinations or grossly disorganized behavior consistent with DSM-III criteria [American Psychiatric Association 1980]); 2) *Conflict* group, adolescents who were not psychotic and who were engaged in interpersonal conflict (argument or dispute) with the victim; and 3) *Crime* group, adolescents who committed the homicide in the course of another crime, such as a robbery or rape. Information concerning the adolescent's prior adjustment in several domains was employed as a basis for testing the external validity of the proposed typology.

The Michigan Study of Adolescent Homicide

To identify a comparatively large sample of adolescents who had committed murder, we reviewed case records of the Michigan Center for Forensic Psychiatry for the years 1977 through mid-1985. The Forensic Center is the centralized state facility mandated by law to conduct evaluations of both a defendant's competency to stand trial and criminal responsibility (legal insanity). Each year the Forensic Center conducts approximately 1200–1500 evaluations of defendants from across the state of Michigan. Archival review identified a total of 88 adolescents (18 years or younger at the time of the offense) charged with murder (first or second degree murder, but not manslaughter).

It should be noted that this sample consists only of adolescents referred for pretrial psychiatric evaluation. We estimate that less than one-third of all adolescent homicide cases were referred for evaluation at the Forensic Center. Nevertheless, a court-referred sample is the group of primary concern to the forensic clinician, and 88 cases are enough to contain a very diverse group of youths. The decision to refer a youth for evaluation may involve many different factors. Some defendants may be referred because of a history of psychiatric difficulties or because of unusual behavior at the time of the offense or in interacting with defense counsel. Other defendants may be referred simply because of the youthfulness of the offender and the seriousness of the crime. Court referral practices also may be influenced by unrelated factors, such as the attitudes and preferences of individual judges and attorneys.

Sixteen of the juvenile homicide cases were eliminated because the case record could not be located (3 cases) or because of an excessive amount of missing information (no social history report or other major document) in the record (13 cases), leaving a total of 72 adolescents charged with homicide.

The selection of an appropriate comparison group posed some difficulty. A "normal" or unselected adolescent control group was not satisfactory because group differences might be a function of general delinquency. In contrast, juveniles charged with violent crimes other than homicide might differ relatively little from those charged with homicide, because in some cases it is only a matter of chance that one assault victim dies while another survives. This reasoning led to the selection of adolescents charged with larceny (car theft or breaking and entering) who did not commit a violent act against a person. Thirty-five adolescents charged with larceny were selected from records of other adolescents evaluated over the same time period. It should be noted that this comparison group was intended to represent those adolescents *who were referred for evaluation* and not the larger group of *all* adolescents charged with larceny.

Data Available for Analysis

The pretrial evaluations were conducted either by a doctoral-level clinical psychologist or board-certified psychiatrist. All examiners had postdegree training in forensic psychology or psychiatry, and all were experienced members of the Forensic Center staff. Records generally included extensive information for each adolescent defendant: 1) police and other investigative reports, including a review of the homicide and relevant evidence, coroner's report, accounts of witnesses, interviews with family and associates of both the victim and defendant, and transcripts of any statements made by the defendant; 2) background information regarding the defendant, including school records, previous mental health records, and reports of previous contacts with juvenile authorities; 3) Forensic Center reports concerning the defendant's competency to stand trial, criminal responsibility, and juvenile status, as requested by the court; 4) Forensic Center reports detailing the defendant's clinical presentation, mental status, social history, and performance on psychological testing; 5) Forensic Center reports of interviews with the defendant's family members or other relevant witnesses, if any; and 6) reports of evaluations by private practitioners working independently of the Forensic Center.

As described elsewhere (Cornell et al. 1987a), data coding was undertaken in several stages, with repeated reliability checks. After training, coder agreement on a sample of 15 cases averaged 91 percent for 61 background or clinical variables employed in this study (range 60 to 100 percent, with only two variables below 80 percent). One coder was blind to the study hypotheses and coded approximately two-thirds of the cases.

Demographic and Background Characteristics

Although the primary focus of this chapter is on distinctions within the homicide group, preliminary analyses contrasted homicide and larceny control groups on demographic and other background variables. Our intent is to provide much more detailed information on a much larger sample of juvenile murderers than has been generally available in previous literature.

Age at time of the offense for subjects in the homicide

TABLE 1. Background characteristics of adolescents charged with homicide or larceny

Background characteristic	No. (%)		Significance test
	Homicide charge ($n = 72$)	Larceny charge ($n = 35$)	
Age at offense			
15 or under	13 (18)	1 (3)	
16	10 (14)	2 (6)	
17	27 (38)	19 (54)	
18	22 (31)	13 (37)	
Mean $\pm$ SD	16.7 $\pm$ 1.28	17.3 $\pm$ 0.71	$t = 2.31$, $p < 0.05$
Race			$p = 0.04$[a]
White	39 (54)	26 (74)	
Nonwhite	33 (46)	9 (26)	
Parent marital status			$\chi^2 = 0.85$, NS
Married	18 (25)	6 (17)	
Divorced	46 (64)	25 (71)	
Never married	8 (11)	4 (11)	
High school status			$p = 0.07$[a]
Enrolled/graduated	37 (51)	12 (34)	
Dropout/expelled	35 (49)	23 (66)	
Mental health treatment			
Outpatient treatment			$p = 0.001$[a]
Yes	16 (22)	19 (54)	
No	56 (78)	16 (46)	
Inpatient treatment			$p = 0.002$[a]
Yes	11 (15)	15 (43)	
No	61 (85)	20 (57)	
Medication used			$p = 0.01$[a]
Yes	8 (11)	11 (31)	
No	64 (89)	24 (69)	

[a] By Fisher exact test.

67

group ranged from 12 to 18 years, with a mean age of 16.7 years. Homicide subjects were significantly younger than larceny control subjects (Table 1). The homicide group also contained a relatively greater proportion of nonwhite subjects.

Relatively few of the adolescents in the homicide group had a history of prior mental health treatment compared to the control group. Control youths were more likely to have had a history of outpatient psychiatric treatment, inpatient psychiatric treatment, and treatment with psychotropic medication.

A second set of analyses contrasted groups in history of delinquent activities before the offense. Almost half of the adolescents in the homicide group had no history of prior arrests, whereas the majority of adolescents in the control group had one or more arrests (Table 2). Also, adolescents in the homicide group were significantly less likely to have a history of placement in a juvenile facility.

TABLE 2. History of delinquency in adolescents charged with homicide or larceny

	No. (%)		
Delinquent behavior	Homicide charge (n=72)	Larceny charge (n=35)	Significance test
Prior arrests			$\chi^2 = 11.74$, p <0.01
None	31 (43)	7 (20)	
One	15 (21)	4 (11)	
Two	12 (17)	7 (20)	
Three or more	14 (19)	17 (49)	
Prior juvenile placements			$p = 0.03$ by Fisher exact test
No	52 (72)	18 (51)	
Yes	20 (28)	17 (49)	
Alcohol abuse			$\chi^2 = 1.87$, NS
No occasional drinking	19 (26)	7 (20)	
Occasional drinking	29 (40)	19 (54)	
Regular/heavy drinking	24 (33)	9 (26)	
Other drug abuse			$\chi^2 = 0.31$, NS
No occasional drug use	15 (21)	7 (20)	
Occasional drug use	28 (39)	12 (34)	
Regular/heavy drug use	29 (40)	16 (46)	

Analysis of Race and Age Differences

In view of the previously mentioned group differences in race and age, further analyses were undertaken to examine any effects these variables might have had on the other results presented in Tables 1 or 2 (see also Cornell et al. 1987a). First, we considered whether there were race differences within the homicide group. There was a significant association between race and parent marital status, with a tendency for greater marital disruption among nonwhites (4 of 33 or 12 percent wed, 70 percent divorced, and 18 percent never married) than among whites (14 of 39 or 36 percent wed, 59 percent divorced, and 5 percent never married). Also, there was significantly more inpatient treatment among whites (9 of 39 or 23 percent) than nonwhites (2 of 33 or 6 percent), $p = 0.04$ by Fisher exact test. No other race analyses within the homicide group were significant. In view of the small number (9 cases) of nonwhites in the control group, similar race analyses were not undertaken.

Next, we repeated homicide versus control group comparisons of the white adolescents. There were significant associations between group status and each of the following: school enrollment, outpatient treatment, and inpatient treatment (all $p < 0.05$ by Fisher exact test). Comparisons for the following variables were no longer significant: medication use, arrest history, and prior juvenile placement. No other analyses of white subjects were significant, and group contrasts were not repeated on nonwhite subjects because of the small number of nonwhite control cases.

Analyses for age were similar to those for race. First, age differences were examined by analyses of variance (ANOVAs) calculated separately for the homicide and control groups. Among homicide cases, age was positively associated with dropping out of school, alcohol use, and drug use. Among control cases, there were no significant age differences.

Group contrasts were repeated on the subgroup of 17–18-year-old subjects as a control for possible age effects. There were significant associations between group status and each of the following: outpatient treatment, inpatient treatment, arrests, and juvenile placement (all $p < 0.05$ by Fisher exact test). No other analyses were significant.

Offense Characteristics

The next series of analyses investigated the circumstances of the offense for adolescents within the homicide group (Table 3). Homicide cases were divided into three groups based on the relationship between the adolescent and his victim: family member, familiar person (friend or acquaintance), or stranger. There were six multiple homicide cases: three involved the murder of at least one family member (classified under family murder) and three involved the murder of strangers.

TABLE 3. Offense characteristics of 72 adolescents charged with homicide

| | No. (%) with victim relationship | | | |
| | Family member (n = 15) | Familiar person (n = 34) | Stranger (n = 23) | |
Offense characteristic				Significance test
Weapon used				$\chi^2 = 19.56$, $p < 0.01$
None	0 (0)	5 (15)	11 (48)	
Gun	9 (60)	9 (26)	6 (26)	
Knife	4 (27)	12 (35)	2 (8)	
Club/other	2 (13)	8 (24)	4 (17)	
Intoxication status[a]				$\chi^2 = 2.76$, NS
Not intoxicated	8 (53)	18 (53)	7 (32)	
Intoxicated	7 (47)	16 (47)	15 (68)	
Accomplice involved				$\chi^2 = 13.87$, $p < 0.0$
Yes	3 (20)	7 (21)	15 (65)	
No	12 (80)	27 (79)	8 (35)	
Sex of victim[b]				$\chi^2 = 1.68$, NS
Male	9 (75)	19 (56)	11 (52)	
Female	3 (25)	15 (44)	10 (48)	
Sexual assault				$\chi^2 = 4.79$, $p < 0.10$
Yes	0 (0)	5 (15)	6 (26)	
No	15 (100)			

[a] Intoxication status unknown for one case in the stranger group.
[b] Five cases of multiple homicide involving both a male and a female victim were omitted from this analysis.

For ease of presentation, offense characteristics for each of the three groups will be described separately, along with illustrative material taken from case files. Adolescents who murdered family members most often did so with a gun, and none of them failed to use some kind of weapon. About half were intoxicated on drugs or alcohol, and most acted without an accomplice. Excluding double homicides involving both a male and female victim, most victims were male and none were sexually assaulted. Of the 15 cases involving murder of a family member, relative victims included nine fathers (one a stepfather), four mothers, one brother, one aunt, and two uncles (one a custodial parent and the other age 12 years). In two of these cases, an adolescent killed both his mother and father. In another case, an adolescent killed his father, his father's girlfriend, his own girlfriend, and a neighbor who attempted to intervene.

The adolescents who murdered a familiar person constituted the largest and most varied group. The most commonly used weapon was a knife, approximately half of the adolescents were intoxicated, and most acted alone. The majority of victims were male, but 5 of the 15 female victims were sexually assaulted. Motives for the offense were diverse, but generally fell into two broad categories. Some of the adolescents murdered in the course of an argument, recent dispute, or ongoing conflict with the victim. Others murdered in the course of another criminal act, such as burglary or rape. Examples of the former include a youth who murdered a male rival for his girlfriend, and a youth who murdered a female peer who had constantly teased and belittled him in front of others. Adolescents who murdered familiar persons in the course of another crime included numerous youths who were caught burglarizing a neighbor's home and several who raped a female acquaintance.

Adolescents who murdered a stranger most often used no weapon other than their hands. This might be associated with the fact that most of these adolescents acted with an accomplice who may have assisted in overpowering the victim. The majority of adolescents were intoxicated. Most of these youths murdered in the course of another criminal act. Several of them committed sexual assaults; others were engaged in robbery or burglary of the victim. One adolescent habitually went out with a friend to beat up vagrants for no apparent motive other than the act of aggression itself. There were three multiple homicides, two involving the murder of a man and a woman, and one involving the murder of two men.

Although there is value in classifying homicides on the basis of the victim relationship, the large number of victims who were familiar persons to the youth (that is, neither relatives nor strangers) poses a problem. These cases are sufficiently diverse that some additional distinction seems necessary. It seems important to distinguish homicides associated with the robbery or rape of the familiar person from those associated with an argument or dispute.

Typology of Juvenile Murderers

In the next stage of data coding, two of us (D.C. and E.B.) independently classified the 72 homicide cases into the three subgroups described earlier: psychotic, conflict, or crime. Coders were limited to information concerning the offense itself (versions provided by police report and defendant's statement to the forensic examiner) and did not have access to background information used in the second stage of coding. Each coder independently classified all 72 cases, with 89 percent agreement ($\kappa = 0.80$).

Classification of the 72 adolescents yielded the following distribution: 1) psychotic—5 cases (7 percent); 2) conflict—30 cases (42 percent); and 3) crime—37 cases (51 percent). Descriptive information concerning the circumstances of the offense is presented in Table 4. It should be noted that offense information is not independent of group classification, because that information was available to coders in making group assignments. For this reason, data are presented only for descrip-

TABLE 4. Descriptive information concerning 72 adolescent homicides

Descriptive information	No. (%)		
	Crime group (n=37)	Conflict group (n=30)	Psychotic group (n=5)[a]
Victim relationship			
Family member	1 (3)	13 (43)	1
Familiar person	15 (41)	15 (50)	2
Stranger	21 (57)	2 (7)	2
Weapon used			
None	13 (35)	2 (7)	1
Gun	9 (24)	14 (47)	1
Knife	7 (19)	8 (27)	3
Club/other	8 (22)	6 (20)	0
Intoxication			
Alcohol/drugs	27 (73)[b]	9 (30)	2
None reported	9 (24)	21 (70)	3
Accomplice present			
Yes	21 (57)	4 (13)	0
No	16 (43)	26 (87)	5
Posthomicide behavior			
Fled scene	36 (97)	19 (63)	3
Arrested at scene	1 (3)	11 (37)	2

[a] Due to small sample size, percentages not presented.
[b] In one case, information about intoxication status was missing.

tive purposes, to elaborate differences among adolescent groups in the circumstances of the homicide.

Prior Adjustment Characteristics

The purpose of the final series of data analyses was to investigate the adolescents' prior adjustment. Data coding for these comparisons began by clustering 52 prior adjustment variables into eight composite categories: family dysfunction, school adjustment, childhood problems, violence history, delinquent behavior, substance abuse, psychiatric problems, and stressful life events before the offense. The development of these categories has been described elsewhere (Cornell et al. 1987b). Composite variables, items, and weights are reported in Table 5.

Table 5. Individual items and weights comprising composite variables

Composite variable (weight)	Items
Family dysfunction (.54)	Parent marital status (0-married, 1-divorced/separated, 2-never wed) Father absence (0-none, 1-one year +, 2-absent since age 5) Mother absence (same as father absence) Stepparent conflict (0-no, 1-yes) Spouse abuse (0-no, 2-yes) Child abuse (0-no, 3-yes) Parent substance abuse (0-no, 1-one parent, 2-two parents) Parent psychiatric hospitalization (0-no, 1-one parent, 2-two parents)
School adjustment (.52)	Status at offense (0-enrolled/graduated, 2-dropout/expelled) Grades (0-average or above, 2-below average) Special Education placement (0-no, 1-yes) School behavior problems (0-no, 1-non-assaultive, 2-assaultive) Truancy (0-no, 1-yes) Suspensions 0-no, 1-yes)
Childhood problems (preteen) (.58)	Birth defect/delivery problem (0-no, 1-yes) Serious illness (0-no, 1-yes) Diagnosed hyperactive (0-no, 1-yes, 2-on medication) Other symptoms (1 per symptom: seizures, enuresis, mild retardation, tantrums, etc.)
Violence history (.44)	Assaulted adults (0-no, 1-one time, 2-two +) Assaulted peers (0-no, 1-one time, 2-two +) Injured someone (0-no, 1-yes) Destroyed property (0-no, 1-yes) Cruelty to animals (0-no, 1-yes)

Category	Items
Criminal activity (.70)	Auto theft (0-no, 1-one, 2-two +)
	Breaking and entering (0-no, 1-one, 2-two +)
	Shoplifting (0-no, 1-one, 2-two +)
	Arrest record (0-no, 2-one, 3-two, 4-three +)
	Placement in juvenile facility (0-no, 1-one or <one year, 2-two or >1 year)
Substance abuse (.79)	Alcohol use (0-none, 1-some, 2-heavy/severe)
	Drug use (0-none, 1-some, 2-heavy/severe)
	Drug types (0-none, 1-one/two, 2-three/four, 3-five +)
	Drug/alcohol charge (0-none, 1-one, 2-two +)
	Onset of substance use (0-none, 1-age 16 +, 2-13–15, 3-preteen)
	Treatment for substance abuse (0-no, 1-yes)
Psychiatric history (.66)	Previous outpatient treatment (0-no, 1-yes)
	Previous hospitalization (0-no, 1-yes)
	Previous medication (0-no, 1-yes)
	Suicide attempts (0-no, 1-yes)
Stressful life events prior to offense (.36)	Parent conflict (0-no, 1-yes)
	Peer conflict (0-no, 1-yes)
	Bad news/misfortune (0-no, 1-yes)
	Anticipated life change (0-no, 1-yes)
	Other stress (0-no, 1-yes)

Note: Value in parentheses after each item is alpha coefficient.

After training, interrater reliability (Pearson correlation coefficient) for composite variable scores ranged from $r = 0.74$ to $r = 0.97$, with a mean $r = 0.91$. Coding of composite variables was completed on sections of the five-page abstract that omitted any reference to the defendant's charge, circumstances of the offense, or clinical opinions of the forensic examiner. One coder was blind to the hypotheses of the study (and uninformed that the study concerned adolescent homicide), and this coder's scores for all 107 cases were used in the analyses.

The presence of overall significant differences among the three homicide subgroups and the larceny control group was established first by a multivariate analysis of variance. Further analyses consisted of a series of one-way ANOVAs on each of the eight composite variables. Each ANOVA contained three planned comparisons: 1) larceny control versus homicide; 2) psychotic versus nonpsychotic (crime and conflict); and 3) crime versus conflict.

Overall, the three series of planned comparisons tested 24 hypotheses, 10 of which resulted in statistically significant findings. Control group adolescents scored significantly higher (more problems) than homicide group adolescents on school adjustment, childhood symptoms, criminal activity, and psychiatric history. Within the homicide group, the psychotic adolescents scored significantly higher than the nonpsychotic (crime and conflict) adolescents on psychiatric history, but scored lower on criminal activity. Finally, among the nonpsychotic homicide cases, the crime subgroup scored significantly higher than the conflict subgroup on school adjustment, criminal activity, and substance abuse, but scored lower on stressful life events before the offense. When comparisons were repeated controlling for age and race by analyses of covariance, there was no change in the pattern of significant results.

Given the significant results in the ANOVA planned comparisons, the composite variables were employed in discriminant function analyses to classify adolescents into groups. This specific application of discriminant analysis is not meant for

Table 6. Comparison of adolescent groups on composite background measures

Composite Measures		Homicide			Planned Comparison F Statistic		
	(1) Larceny control Mean (SD) ($n = 35$)	(2) Psychosis Mean (SD) ($n = 5$)	(3) Crime Mean (SD) ($n = 37$)	(4) Conflict Mean (SD) ($n = 30$)	Control (1)[a] vs. homicide (2-3-4)	Psychotic (2)[b] vs. nonpsychotic (3-4)	Crime (3)[b] vs. conflict (4)
Family dysfunction	4.74(3.3)	4.60(4.0)	4.02(2.8)	4.80(3.3)	0.13	0.02	1.00
School adjustment problems	5.37(2.4)	4.00(3.1)	5.54(1.8)	3.10(2.5)	4.67*	0.10	19.77***
Childhood symptoms	1.06(1.4)	0.40(.55)	.73(1.1)	0.33(.66)	4.72*	0.07	2.18
Violence	1.29(1.6)	2.20(1.9)	2.00(1.5)	1.57(1.4)	3.01	0.34	1.32
Criminal activity	5.17(3.0)	0.60(1.3)	3.89(3.2)	2.40(2.0)	16.10***	3.38*	4.13*
Substance abuse	5.46(3.2)	3.80(2.6)	6.27(2.6)	4.37(3.8)	0.71	1.05	5.89**
Psychiatric history	2.06(1.8)	2.80(2.8)	0.65(1.1)	0.50(.55)	4.46*	10.75***	0.17
Stress events prior to offense	0.63(.81)	0.60(.55)	0.76(.86)	1.73(1.1)	3.4	2.3	18.91***

Note: Overall MANOVA F (24, 279) = 4.68, $p < 0.001$.
[a] two-tailed significance tests.
[b] one-tailed significance tests.
*$p < 0.05$ **$p < 0.01$ ***$p < 0.001$

predictive purposes, but is applied descriptively in order to demonstrate the lack of overlap between groups (Huberty 1984). This is one means of verifying that results that are *statistically* significant also indicate more meaningful differences among the individuals comprising each group.

Analyses were conducted by the Michigan Interactive Data Analysis System (MIDAS) DISCRIMINANT program (Fox and Guire 1976), a nonstepwise procedure. The first analysis classified subjects into either the homicide group or larceny control group. Eighty-three (78 percent) of 107 cases were correctly classified. This included correct classification of 26 control and 57 homicide cases; 9 controls were misclassified as homicide cases and 15 homicide cases were misclassified as controls. Using the maximum chance criterion reported by Huberty (1984), the 78 percent classification accuracy was significantly better than the 67.3 percent (72 of 107) accuracy expected by chance, $z = 2.26$, $p < 0.05$.

The second discriminant function analysis was limited to classifying subjects in the crime and conflict groups. This analysis correctly classified 55 (82 percent) of 67 cases, including correct classification of 32 crime and 23 conflict cases and misclassification of 5 crime and 7 conflict cases. The overall 82 percent accuracy was significantly better than the 37 (55.2 percent) of 67 cases that could be classified using the maximum chance criterion, $z = 5.73$, $p < 0.001$.

Implications

These results permit a much more differentiated view of adolescent homicide than has been possible in the past—both in comparing adolescent homicide defendants with other adolescents referred for pretrial evaluation and in distinguishing subtypes within the homicide group. In the present sample, adolescents charged with the nonviolent offense of larceny scored higher (more problems) on composite measures of school adjustment, childhood symptoms, criminal activity, and psychiatric history. These adolescents should *not* be construed as representative of all delinquents charged with larceny, but instead of the more select subset who are referred for pretrial evaluation. From the standpoint of the mental health professional conducting evaluations for the court, this would seem to be the more relevant comparison group.

It is noteworthy that adolescents charged with the far more serious crime of homicide have relatively less troubled backgrounds. In part, this may reflect a greater tendency to refer homicide defendants for pretrial evaluation because of the seriousness of the offense, even in the absence of background factors (such as previous psychiatric treatment) that might support pursuing an insanity defense.

Perhaps the most surprising finding was that so few of the homicide group adolescents were classified as psychotic at the time of the offense. Based on extensive information obtained in the course of pretrial evaluations, only five adolescents (7 percent) had psychotic symptoms in accord with DSM-III criteria. This finding runs counter to case reports and theoretical contention that many juvenile murderers are psychotic (Lewis 1981; Sadoff 1971; Satten et al. 1960; Sendi and Blomgren 1975). Such claims could be a reflection of limited samples drawn from clinical practice or general psychiatric settings. Other reports (Hellsten and Katila 1965; Walshe-Brennan 1977; Zenoff and Zients 1979; for others, see Chapter 1) have found a low incidence or absence of psychotic adolescents in their samples. Based on a general (primarily adult) sample of 43 homicide defendants referred for insanity evaluation, Kahn (1971) reported that only 6 were diagnosed as psychotic.

The adolescents in the crime and conflict groups were distinguished on the basis of different apparent motives for the offense. Additional information in Table 4 elaborates the circumstances of the offense. Crime group adolescents tended to murder strangers and some familiar persons (for example, neighbors, acquaintances) but rarely family members. They most often used no weapon and over half had an accomplice (who may have assisted in overpowering the victim). Three-quarters of these adolescents were intoxicated on alcohol or drugs at the time of the offense, and all but one fled the scene. In contrast, conflict group adolescents most often murdered family members or familiar persons. They most often acted alone and almost always used a weapon, most frequently a gun. Less than one-third were intoxicated, and over one-third were arrested at the scene of the offense.

These differences between homicide subtypes are not independent of group classification and have only descriptive value. External evidence of the validity of the typology must be derived from factors unrelated to the circumstances of the offense. Compared to the conflict group, adolescents in the crime group presented a much more consistent history of prior delinquent behavior, such as committing breaking and entering and other offenses that lead to being placed in juvenile facilities. They have more extensive histories of school problems, such as truancy, failing grades, and dropping out. Although the amount of substance abuse was generally high in both groups, crime group youths had relatively greater problems. Finally, crime group youths reported a lower frequency of stressful life events before the offense than did youths in the conflict group.

Implications for Research on Violent Behavior

The existence of distinct subtypes of homicidal adolescents, if supported by further research, would have direct implications for research on the etiology of adolescent violence. Current conceptions of adolescent violence alternatively emphasize the etiological role of genetic, neuropsychological, social learning, or psychodynamic factors (Keith 1984; Lewis 1981). In the present sample, adolescents grouped according to the circumstances in which they exhibited extreme violent behavior differed consistently in composite measures of prior adjustment. These results suggest developmental differences among violent adolescents and raise the possibility of distinguishable developmental pathways to violent behavior.

These findings have special relevance for research on the

80

clinical prediction of violent behavior. Much of this research attempts to identify "risk factors" (such as features in the individual's background) that are associated with subsequent violent behavior (Monahan 1981). However, the present study demonstrates that even the most violent behavior can be exhibited by adolescents with very different prior adjustment histories. Research on the predictions of violent behavior may be seriously impaired by failure to differentiate among the motivational circumstances of violent behavior and should recognize the possibility of distinct sets of risk factors appropriate to different circumstances.

Forensic Implications

If supported by additional research, the proposed typology could have implications for future treatment and disposition of juvenile homicide defendants. Currently, Michigan statutes, as well as laws in most other states, provide for waiver of juveniles into the adult court system (Smith et al. 1980). Juvenile waiver criteria commonly include, among other factors, consideration of the adolescent's psychological adjustment and amenability to treatment. Adolescents in the crime group might be regarded as the most maladjusted with respect to character or the most antisocial in orientation, a factor that could support waiver into adult court (Zenoff and Zients 1979).

Adolescents in the conflict group might be less maladjusted and more amenable to treatment, factors that could support a decision to retain juvenile court jurisdiction of the case. Special caution is indicated regarding implications for adolescents in the psychotic group because there are so few cases, but presumably these adolescents are most in need of treatment in a psychiatric setting and may be legitimate candidates for an insanity defense.

Reasoning along similar lines, Zenoff and Zients (1979) describe seven cases of "nonempathic" murderers who killed strangers in the course of a robbery or for no apparent reason.

They concluded that these adolescents are at greater risk for future violent and/or delinquent behavior and should be treated differently by the court system than six adolescents they identified as having murdered an acquaintance in the course of an argument. Follow-up studies of juvenile murderers eventually released to the community or seen in long-term psychotherapy lend some support to this view (Cormier and Markus 1980; Hellsten and Katila 1965; Scherl and Mack 1966).

References

Adams K: The child who murders. Criminal Justice and Behavior 1:51–61, 1974

American Psychiatric Association: Diagnostic and Statistical Manual of Mental Disorders, Third Edition. Washington, DC, American Psychiatric Association, 1980

Bender L: Children and adolescents who have killed. Am J Psychiatry 116:510–513, 1959

Bender L, Curran F: Children and adolescents who kill. Journal of Criminal Psychopathology 1:296–322, 1940

Corder B, Ball B, Haizlip T, et al: Adolescent parricide: a comparison with other adolescent murder. Am J Psychiatry 133:957–961, 1976

Cormier B, Markus B: A longitudinal study of adolescent murderers. Bull Am Acad Psychiatry Law 8:240–260, 1980

Cormier B, Angliker C, Gagne P, et al: Adolescents who kill members of the family, in Family Violence: An International and Interdisciplinary Study. Edited by Eekelaar J, Katz S. Toronto, Butterworth, 1978

Cornell D, Benedek E, Benedek D: Characteristics of adolescents charged with homicide: review of 72 cases. Behavioral Sciences and the Law 5:11–23, 1987a

Cornell D, Benedek E, Benedek D: Juvenile homicide: prior adjustment and a proposed typology. Am J Orthopsychiatry 57:383–393, 1987b

Duncan J, Duncan G: Murder in the family: a study of some homicidal adolescents. Am J Psychiatry 127:74–78, 1971

Fox D, Guire K: Documentation for MIDAS, 3rd edition. Ann Arbor, Statistical Research Laboratory, The University of Michigan, 1976

Hellsten P, Katila O: Murder and other homicide by children under 15 in Finland. Psychiatric Q Suppl 39:54–74, 1965

Huberty C: Issues in the use and interpretation of discriminant analyses. Psychol Bull 95:156–171, 1984

Kahn M: Murderers who plead insanity: a descriptive factor-analytic study of personality, social and history variables. Genetic Psychology Monographs 84:275–360, 1971

Keith C: The Aggressive Adolescent: Clinical Perspectives. New York, The Free Press, 1984

Lewis D: Vulnerabilities to Delinquency. Jamaica, NY, Spectrum Publications, 1981

McCarthy J: Narcissism and the self in homicidal adolescents. Am J Psychoanal 38:19–29, 1978

Megargee E: The prediction of violence with psychological tests, in Current Topics in Clinical and Community Psychology. Edited by Spielberg C. New York, Academic Press, 1970

Monahan J: The Clinical Prediction of Violent Behavior. Rockville, MD, U.S. Department of Health and Human Services, 1981

Olweus D: Familial and temperamental determinants of aggressive behavior in adolescent boys: a causal analysis. Developmental Psychology 16:644–660 1980

Roth L (ed): Clinical Treatment of the Violent Person. Rockville, MD, Department of Health and Human Services, Publication No. (ADM) 85-1425, 1985

Sadoff R: Clinical observations on parricide. Psychiatric Q 45:65–69, 1971

Sargent S: Children who kill—a family conspiracy? Social Work 7:35–42, 1962

Satten J, Menninger K, Rosen I, et al: Murder without apparent motive: a study in personality disorganization. Am J Psychiatry 117:18–53, 1960

Scherl D, Mack J: A study of adolescent matricide. J Am Acad Child Psychiatry 5:559–593, 1966

Sendi I, Blomgren P: A comparative study of predictive criteria in the predisposition of homicidal adolescents. Am J Psychiatry 132:423–428, 1975

Smith C, Alexander P, Kemp G, et al: Reports of the National Juvenile Justice Assessment Centers: Vol. III: Legislation, Jurisdiction, Program Interventions, and Confidentiality of Juvenile Records. Washington, DC, U.S. Department of Justice, National Institute for Juvenile Justice and Delinquency Prevention, 1980

Solway K, Richardson L, Hays J, et al: Adolescent murderers: literature review and preliminary research findings, in Violence and the Violent Individual. Edited by Hays J, Roberts T, Solway K. New York, SP Medical and Scientific Books, 1981

Walshe-Brennan K: A socio-psychological investigation of young murderers. British Journal of Criminology 17:58–63, 1977

Wolfgang M, Figlio R, Sellin T: Delinquency in a Birth Cohort. Chicago, University of Chicago Press, 1972

Zenoff E, Zients A: Juvenile murderers: should the punishment fit the crime? International Journal of Law and Psychiatry 2:533–553, 1979

Chapter 4

The Adolescent Witness to Homicide

SPENCER ETH, M.D.

Chapter 4

The Adolescent Witness to Homicide

*T*he enormity of the problem of juvenile homicide is apparent throughout this volume. Murder is the fastest growing cause of death in the United States, and adolescents are well represented as both perpetrators and victims (Schetky 1985). Clearly, attention is appropriately focused on the deceased and his or her surviving family, and on the assailant. However, in the grim aftermath of a homicide it is common to overlook the plight of those persons who were directly exposed to the violence. It is the contention of this chapter that the witnesses to homicide include a sizable population of adolescents who are themselves at high risk for developing significant symptomatology and yet are quite responsive to psychiatric intervention.

Perspectives on Homicide

Each of the more than 20,000 homicides committed annually in the United States sets into motion its own emotional chain of events. Present at the incident are the victim, the perpetrator, and the eyewitnesses. The victim suffers the premature termination of his or her life, whereas the perpetrator, if apprehended, faces the full weight of the criminal justice system. The consequences for the eyewitnesses are legion and will be considered in detail in the pages that follow. The emotional repercussions do not end with these persons physically present at the scene of the crime. The police, who are invariably summoned, are themselves affected by viewing the carnage of a homicide. Police officers are then dispatched to inform the deceased's family of the unexpected passing of their loved one. This task of death notification has been shown to be enormously stressful for the police (Eth et al. 1987). Officers feel unprepared to deal with the grief and anger evoked in the victims' families and are concerned with the danger of an attack directed against them as the bearers of bad news. Homicide duty may be a major contributor to the prevalence of occupational burnout found in urban police forces.

News of the violent death catapults the surviving family into profound grief. Homicide is always sudden and unexpected and confers a high risk of pathological mourning. In a study of young widows, the group with the least warning experienced intense shock, severe separation anxiety, and confused feelings of anger and guilt. Contending with this type of death may represent the greatest challenge most people will encounter in their lives (Parkes and Weiss 1983). As word of the homicide spreads, other relatives, friends, and neighbors are affected. The ripple effect can even extend into the classroom of a child whose parent or sibling was killed. The classmates discover that the intrusion of actual violence into their school community contrasts starkly with the thousands of simulated acts of mayhem they have seen on television. Many of these children respond with anxiety over their heightened sense of vulnerability, and they may exhibit behavioral disturbances that interfere with the educational process. Specific group interventions have been described that can assist school staff and children in coping with the stress following a violent occurrence (Eth et al. 1985).

Adolescent Exposure

Homicide, the killing of one person by another, has emerged as a public health problem of major proportions (Morbidity and Mortality Weekly Report 1986). Since the mid-1950s the risk of homicide in the city of Los Angeles has increased sixfold. During the last decade the overall homicide rate was 17.1/100,000/year; for Hispanics and blacks the rates were 2.3 and

5.6 times greater. Black men between the ages of 25 and 34 years had a homicide rate of 143/100,000/year. Homicide is now the second leading cause of teenage fatality in the United States, accounting for about 13.5 percent of all deaths in this age group (Blum 1987). In 1985, about 600 homicides were committed in the city of Detroit alone. An examination of the police records of half of these cases revealed that in 52 homicides, 136 children were clearly identified as eyewitnesses to the crimes (Judy Roth, personal communication). Of these witnesses 56 percent were male, 92 percent were black, and 80 percent were teenagers. In 31 percent of the homicides witnessed by adolescents the victim was a family member, in 21 percent the perpetrator was a family member, and in 48 percent neither the deceased nor the killer was a relative of the young witness. These statistics underscore the tragedy of this epidemic of preventable deaths among otherwise healthy young adults. Further, the data confirm that adolescents are routine observers of homicide. The impact of violence on these young eyewitnesses is a matter of great concern to the mental health professions and society alike.

Two major factors figure prominently in shaping the adolescent's responses to lethal violence. The first factor covers the specific details of the homicides, whereas the second involves the characteristics of the witness, including the developmental issues of adolescence. There are an inexhaustible variety of possible circumstances for a homicide. Nevertheless, these crimes may be categorized along certain useful guidelines, such as the relationships of the persons involved. From the perspective of the adolescent witness, the perpetrator and victim must fall into one of the following groups: relatives, acquaintances, or strangers. The more intense the emotional relationship the witness has with the victim and perpetrator, the more serious the consequences. Similarly, the type of homicide exerts a powerful influence in determining the range of psychological outcomes for the adolescent witness. People are killed by others in the context of domestic disputes, crimes, gang violence, warfare, and by accident. Each of these situations generates its own interplay of psychological themes. For example, an adolescent may observe an argument between parents escalate to murderous rage. The offspring will experience feelings of grief for the slain parent and ambivalence for the surviving parent, while contending with conflicts over guilt and aggression. For the adolescent soldier, combat against an unknown enemy challenges the intrapsychic processes of moral development and impulse control.

The adolescent witness to homicide brings to that situation a personal history that uniquely defines the experience. Knowledge of the persons involved and the type of killing may suggest a certain intensity and meaning for the event but can never foretell precisely how that adolescent will react. The response to a psychosocial stressor is a function of an individual's appraisal of the situation and capacity to process, understand, and incorporate it into a belief system (Rutter 1985). These operations reflect the adolescent's self-esteem and self-efficacy; temperament and personality; cognitive, interpersonal, and behavioral repertoire; and range of social competence and problem-solving skills. The product of all of these internal variables is constantly changing while simultaneously interacting with the external environment. Bender (1959) proposed that the reaction to homicide is commensurate with the adolescent's previous psychiatric diagnosis and level of integration of family and community. A quarter century later, Eth and Pynoos (1985a) speculated that susceptibility of a particular child to psychic trauma is determined jointly by the content and intensity of the event and by the child's genetic, constitutional, and personality makeup; past life experiences; and state of mind and phase of development.

Adolescence

There are about 36 million Americans between the ages of 10 and 19 years, of whom 15 percent are black, 9 percent are Hispanic, and 18 percent are impoverished. This period of human life, between childhood and adulthood, has been a source of bewilderment from at least the time of Hesiod in the 8th century B.C. ("the present youth are exceedingly wise and impatient of restraint"). The passage from a state of familial dependence to worldly freedom has similarly mystified psychologists since Hall coined the term adolescence in 1904. How do children come to be emancipated from their homes to work and love independently? Surely the mental processes of adolescence must be as dramatic and complex as the concomitant physical changes of puberty. Traditional wisdom has held that adolescence is "a time of crisis, often of great crisis" (Group for the Advancement of Psychiatry 1968, p. 101). Early psychoanalysts had depicted adolescence as characterized by a lowering of ego strength coupled with an upsurge of aggressive and sexual impulses (Freud 1958). The result of these forces is a disruption of psychic equilibrium and ubiquitous, though transient, psychiatric symptomatology. The extant empirical data, however, suggest otherwise (Oldham 1978). Psychopathology is not a normative feature of adolescence, but may indicate a diagnosable disorder that in the absence of appropriate treatment can disrupt the developmental processes of adolescence and progress to adult disturbance.

One form of psychopathology that commonly afflicts adolescents is traumatization by a catastrophic psychosocial stressor. Psychic trauma, in addition to producing enduring symptoms, can interfere with the salient tasks of this phase of life, particularly cognitive and moral development. The teenage years embrace a widening scope of intellectual activity that prominently features an increased awareness and capability for insight and self-judgment. About a third of adolescents attain a Piagetian level of formal operational thought, and its related postconventional morality reflects a grasp of abstract concepts and an ability to reason from different perspectives. Cognitive maturation provides an antidote to the egocentricity and selfishness that contribute to the unsavory reputation of this age group. Rational thought also extends the boundaries of control over affects, impulses, and behavior underlying the capacity for independent living.

Erikson (1963) selected "identity versus role confusion" as the normative crisis of adolescence, emphasizing the critical importance of the emergence of a unique and coherent character. Integrity of the adolescent's personality may itself depend on the establishment of stable, clearly defined self and object representations freed from the emotional entanglements of early family life. In fact, Anna Freud believed that the primary work of adolescence is negotiating the difficult separation from incestuous object ties (Eth 1983). Thus, this delicate and complicated process of the transformation of child into adult can be adversely affected in many ways by psychic trauma.

Post-Traumatic Stress Disorder

Post-traumatic stress disorder (PTSD) refers to that cluster of symptoms that characteristically appears after an extremely disturbing life event outside of the range of usual human experience. Although the early literature linked the development of this syndrome to brain injury, it is now accepted that the etiology is psychogenic, and the condition is accordingly classified among the anxiety disorders. The specific term PTSD is relatively new, having first appeared in DSM-III in 1980 (American Psychiatric Association 1980). However, conditions that would be identified as PTSD have been described for over a century under a variety of names (that is, shell shock, survivor syndrome, gross stress reaction, fright hysteria, traumatic neurosis, and stress response syndrome).

PTSD is included in DSM-III-R, the current revision of DSM-III (American Psychiatric Association 1987). Although in general DSM-III-R avoids etiological assumptions, for PTSD there is the clear implication that the psychosocial stressor has provoked the illness insofar as that trauma would have elicited significant distress in almost everyone. DSM-III-R lists as a specific example of an appropriate stressor the experience of seeing another person killed by physical violence and notes that the resulting symptoms are apparently more severe and long-lasting when the traumatic event is of human design.

In addition to the existence of the recognizable stressor, DSM-III-R diagnostic criteria for PTSD require the presence for at least one month of certain symptoms from three groups. The first group involves re-experiencing the event through intrusive memories, recurrent dreams, flashbacks, and anniversary reactions. The second group of symptoms pertains to the persistent avoidance of associated stimuli or numbing of responsiveness as evidenced by thought and activity avoidance, psychogenic amnesia, affective and cognitive dulling, interpersonal detachment, and pessimistic expectation of the future. The final group of typical findings includes symptoms of increased arousal indicated by sleep disturbance, irritability, hypervigilance, and exaggerated autonomic reactions. Although this organization of the diagnostic criteria is new to DSM-III-R, the symptoms themselves for the most part were listed in DSM-III. The usefulness of that PTSD construct was confirmed in a study of 66 outpatients evaluated after a serious life event. About three-fourths of these adult patients reported the presence of typical symptoms regardless of age, sex, and personality type (Horowitz et al. 1980).

Children and adolescents are by no means immune to the psychopathological impact of traumatic events, despite a relative paucity of literature on this age group. DSM-III-R reflects our current understanding that youngsters may exhibit the classic symptoms of PTSD as listed. In addition, other characteristics of PTSD have been identified as common in children. These phenomena include increased misperception of the duration and sequencing of time and events, retrospective presifting or premonition formation, reenactment or the unknowing performance of acts similar to the traumatic occurrence, marked and possibly enduring personality alterations, and changes in the recognition and tolerance of the affect of fear, contributing to inhibition or counter-phobic behavior (Eth and Pynoos 1985a). In contrast to adults, children do not report stress-induced amnesia or disbelief about the reality of what they had experienced, although they may produce fantasies as a means to undo the traumatic event and reverse its consequences. Considering both the DSM-III-R criteria and these child-specific symptoms, it is apparent that PTSD can produce deleterious effects on cognition (including memory, school performance, and learning), affect, interpersonal relations, impulse control, behavior, autonomic function, and symptom formation.

Clinical Evaluation

The adolescent recently exposed to homicide may be withdrawn, distressed, or uncooperative, making direct questioning about the traumatic event difficult for the clinician. Pynoos and Eth (1986) have detailed a three-stage, semistructured interview protocol that facilitates a spontaneous and complete exploration of the child's subjective experiences while permitting support and closure within a two-hour time frame. This technique is especially useful for the adolescent witness to homicide.

Prior to meeting with the adolescent, the therapist attempts to collect information from the referring source about the circumstances of the event and the adolescent's response and current situation. It is useful to begin the session by asking the adolescent to draw a picture and tell a story about whatever comes to mind. This standard art therapy gambit serves as a convenient "icebreaker" that even the most resistant youth finds difficult to refuse (Landgarten 1981). The quality of the work itself varies considerably in style and content; its importance, however, derives from the therapeutic value of turning the passive experience of witness into the active process of artistic creation and from the projective meaning of the product (Wohl and Kaufman 1985). It is assumed that the traumatic incident will be represented in some form in the picture or story, and that this reference will provide the key that allows the clinician to open the adolescent to direct discussion about the trauma.

The second stage of the interview is marked by the transition from the drawing and story to the actual event through an interpretation by the therapist. A statement such as: "I suppose that you wish you were on vacation far away from the violence in your neighborhood like the girl in your drawing" and "I wonder if you feel that knowing first aid like the boy in your story would have saved your friend's life" are examples of comments that may enable the adolescent to verbalize the emotional pain associated with psychic trauma. The therapist must be prepared to offer comfort and support as the patient contends with the intensity of affect and ideation. The act of re-experiencing and sharing the trauma in the controlled safety of a session is inherently therapeutic and should not be avoided.

After the adolescent has obtained some relief from the emotional outcry, the therapist should assist in a systematic re-appraisal of the traumatic event. Many witnesses will dwell on the central action of the homicide. Exploration should extend beyond a verbal description of the visual memory to encompass other sensory perceptions, including for instance the sound and smell of gunfire and the concomitant bodily sensations of autonomic arousal. These are the very recollections that can crystallize into the essential symptoms of post-traumatic stress disorder. However, the adolescent's memory is not limited to the central action. Other circumstances and details may be imbued with a powerful traumatic meaning that might have a particular psychodynamic significance. For example, a strong memory of an assailant, a victim, or perhaps even a police officer may indicate a propensity for an identification. Several adult deputy sheriffs have revealed that after witnessing a murder as children they had been greatly reassured by the arrival of a police officer. Of much greater concern is the development of violent behavior as an identification with the aggressor or of masochistic tendencies as an identification with the victim.

A frequent source of terror for the adolescent witness to homicide is the horrifying sight of physical mutilation. The killing of another human being can involve brutal beatings, bloody knifings, or disfiguring gunshot wounds. The visual impact may be unforgettable and may distort for the adolescent the recollection of that individual as an intact person. The therapist should at some point ask what was the worst part of the experience. The most painful moment may involve a memory from earlier in the day, from the violent occurrence, or from the aftermath, and the memory usually incorporates some significant affective exchange with the victim or assailant. One 14-year-old described a moment of intolerable anger when she heard her father shout, "I'm sorry," after shooting her mother.

The act of homicide inevitably raises the issue of human accountability. DSM-III-R notes that "the disorder [PTSD] is apparently more severe and longer lasting when the stressor is of human design" (American Psychiatric Association 1987, p. 248). Adolescents have bemoaned how much easier it would have been to accept a death under natural circumstances. Instead they must face the question of who is responsible. Revenge fantasies as well as fears of counter-retaliation by the perpetrator may be prominent when the victim is well liked and the assailant is a stranger. Preoccupation with these aggressive fantasies can be debilitating to the child when they persist, recur, or threaten impulse control. In a situation of family violence the teenager may be thrown into an intense conflict of loyalty that can be appreciated by observing the effort expended to avoid this painful issue in session. The assignment of responsibility may vary over time and even during the interview and may come to include the youngster. Adolescents may blame themselves for not having done more to prevent the violence, even when in reality they were powerless to affect the outcome. One girl felt terribly guilty for not having treated her mother's lethal stab wounds.

Any discussion of violence implicitly leads to inquiry about the adolescent's handling of anger. It is appropriate to ask what he or she does when angry and whether that has changed since witnessing the killing. Not uncommonly an adolescent will report becoming more irritable, argumentative, or hostile. Some will resort to frank aggression in the year following a homicide. The therapist also should be sensitive to the opposite reaction in a youngster who responds to the sight of violence by becoming passive and inhibited.

Given sufficient rapport, it is instructive to survey the DSM-III-R symptoms of PTSD and the common associated features in children. In particular one can ask about recent dreams, nightmares, and other sleep disturbances. Dreams about one's own death are well documented in traumatized youngsters, and such a dream or a feeling of premature mortality can serve as a bridge to questions about future plans. Within hours after viewing homicide, adolescents have vowed never to marry or have children in such a dangerous world. That, in fact, may come to be a part of the legacy of violent death.

Adolescents also may disclose other violence that they have observed. Unfortunately, repeated exposure to the sight of human aggression rarely results in resistance to trauma. The adolescent refugees from the war-torn countries of Central America, in particular, have observed multiple episodes of bombing, execution, or terrorist attack. Images from these scenes often seem to blur into a continuous montage of terrifying violence (Arroyo and Eth 1985). A goal of the initial session is to help the youngster place the events in sequence and thereby gain some mastery over memory function disrupted by inescapable horror.

The final, closure stage of the interview centers on the sensitive, critical process of terminating the session. One approach is to refocus on the adolescent's present concerns. Many young witnesses to homicide demonstrate a deterioration in school performance related to the effects of intrusive, dysphoric recollections of and associations with the violence; the interference of anxious and depressed mood; and the elaboration of a cognitive style of forgetting analogous to the defense mechanism of denial. George Gardner (1971) also has speculated that certain learning disabilities are the consequence of an experience with violence, although he identifies the cause as an inhibition of aggressive learning behavior. Difficulties in secondary school can severely handicap an educational career and should be addressed promptly.

Violence can result in additional changes in life circumstance for the witness. Notoriety from media coverage may be a source of pride, but more often stigmatizes the adolescent in the eyes of schoolmates and neighbors. Involvement in legal proceedings may have myriad effects and will be discussed in detail later in this chapter. It is useful to review and summarize the entire session. The adolescent will then be in a position to appreciate that his or her responses are understandable, realistic, and common. Acceptance of the traumatic experience and its effects will reverse the alienation and enable the adolescent to accept more willingly the support of others. It is important to emphasize that it was perfectly all right to have felt helpless or afraid during the violence and sad or angry afterwards. It is also appropriate to compliment adolescents on their bravery during the event, if such a compliment is deserved, and in all cases to praise their courage in confronting these issues in session. Their beleaguered self-esteem invariably is lifted by words of reassurance and praise from the therapist.

Before ending the interview one should consider alerting the adolescent to the expected course of a traumatic syndrome. The therapist might comment that however miserable the adolescent is feeling, the symptoms should improve over time and with treatment. A warning about a reactivation of symptoms on the anniversary may be in order. This is a convenient place in the interview to discuss therapeutic options and formulate a treatment plan if indicated. If the adolescent is not given another appointment, he or she should be reminded that a session can be arranged at any time in the future. Remarkably, even a single interview can have a considerable therapeutic impact on the young witness to a recent homicide.

Adolescent Trauma and Grief

The developmental, phase-specific influence and nature of homicidal violence deeply color the adolescent's experience. Clinical evaluations of this population frequently reveal a closure of identity formation precipitated by a premature entrance into adulthood. Common to this group is post-traumatic acting-out behavior characterized by school truancy, precocious sexual activity and promiscuity, substance abuse, and even delinquency. Family members and teachers describe these teenagers as more rebellious and are dismayed by unusual antisocial acts. The easy availability of automobiles and weapons can make a lapse of impulse control or a post-traumatic reenactment life threatening. On the first anniversary of witnessing his father's homicide, an adolescent became enraged and attempted to shoot his mother. Many adolescents explain their illicit drug use as a means to relieve the dysphoria arising from the traumatic event. These acting-out behaviors may be understood as a form of the defense mechanism of turning against the self (Freud 1966), in which self-destructive acts serve to distract the adolescent from anxiety and sadness and expiate guilt associated with the violence.

Some adolescents remain uncooperative, suspicious, and guarded in the interview. These adolescents may feel compelled to critically judge the courage of their own actions while paradoxically feeling reluctant to blame the assailant. Eliciting a full account of the sequence of actions can prove quite helpful in assisting adolescent participants to more accurately place themselves in the chain of events. The therapist should be wary of the egocentric tendency of adolescents to inflate their personal role in the crime despite the discomfort that promotes. Many adolescents have the capacity for abstraction and self-observation that will permit them to objectively assign responsibility and understand the function of the criminal justice system. This cognitive ability also may sensitize adolescents to community stigma and strengthen their resolve not to tempt fate by bringing children into this violent world (Krystal 1978).

Homicide, by definition, is an act resulting in the death of a human being. As such the adolescent witness may, in addition to psychic trauma, suffer grief. Grief is the subjective experience and behavior that occur after an emotionally significant loss. It is now widely accepted that adolescents routinely exhibit a range of grief responses as a function of maturity, personality, and cultural milieu. The tasks of mourning for the adolescent, as for the adult, are to accept the loss through reality testing and tolerate the pain of grief. Depending on the intensity of the relationship with the deceased, the adolescent may feel sad, angry, guilty, lonely, tired, nervous, confused, preoccupied, and/or physically ill. Slowly, there is a withdrawal from the memory of the deceased and an increase of available psychic energy for forging new or stronger relationships. Adolescents are subject to the same disturbances of bereavement that afflict adults, including pathological grief in which the mourner is overwhelmed, resorts to maladaptive behavior, or remains frozen in sadness.

It is axiomatic that trauma caused by witnessing a violent death impairs grief work when the horror over the manner of death interferes with thoughts about the deceased. Eth and Pynoos (1985b) have found that traumatic anxiety is a priority concern that compromises the mourner's ability to attend to the fantasies of the deceased that are integral to the grief process. A possible consequence of difficulty in timely and effective grieving is an aborted response. A 13-year-old's mourning for her 19-year-old murdered sister was delayed for six years until the adolescent reached the same age as her sister when she was killed, at which time her grief was precipitated by an anniversary reaction (Burgess 1975). In most cases the mourning process extends for longer than the acute traumatic syndrome. Hence, as the traumatic anxiety diminishes, grief may intensify. Other traumatic factors contribute to the disruption of normal bereavement as well. Reminiscing, which is essential to the grief process, may be drastically inhibited by the intrusive images of the lethal violence and by traumatic ego constriction and numbing. Open grieving may be stifled by a forced silence imposed on the adolescent by a family stung by social stigma (Lister 1982).

In rare instances the violent death of a close family member will prove overwhelming to the adolescent. The obligatory but unsuccessful efforts at relieving traumatic anxiety can leave the adolescent feeling defeated, alone, and terribly sad. Under these circumstances an otherwise comforting reunion fantasy can seem to invite self-destruction. Anderson (1949) reports an adolescent who was present when his father was killed in a rocket attack. This boy's traumatic grief propelled him to a suicide attempt. Another case of pathological mourning in the literature involved an adolescent whose brother was killed in a drugstore while joking with other teenagers (Volkan 1970).

Accidental Homicide

The typology of juvenile murderers covers a spectrum of possible motivations (Bender 1959). At one extreme is the adolescent who commits "accidental" homicide by killing without the conscious thought of hurting the victim. Foodman and Estrada (1977) speculate that this may be the most common type of homicide perpetrated by adolescents. In a sense, adolescents who kill by accident are witnesses to their homicides, but with the additional burden of being the agent responsible for the resulting death. Case reports in the psychiatric literature support the notion that these adolescents are extremely vulnerable to traumatic grief. For example, Carek and Watson (1964) describe a preadolescent who rapidly developed a deterioration in school performance, withdrawal, irritability, depression, vegetative signs, and suicidal ideation after accidentally killing his brother. Another, slightly older boy also mistakenly shot his brother to death. He too became isolated, depressed, confused, and suicidal. This patient responded favorably to multimodal treatment with an antidepressant (Petti and Wells 1980).

Case Example

Thomas C., 17 years old, was interviewed in juvenile hall a month after shooting his 14-year-old sister in the neck and then burying her in the yard. Thomas's personal history was characterized by a chaotic childhood with several changes in residence after his parents' divorce seven years before. Thomas had received treatment for episodes of affective illness earlier in adolescence and was believed to have been using marijuana and alcohol prior to the incident. Thomas had been extremely close to his sister and, in fact, had been planning to run away with her at the time of the shooting.

During session Thomas refused to speak about the shooting, although he did admit to feeling very sad and guilt ridden. He was often tearful in jail and could not keep himself from ruminating about the shooting. He was haunted by nightmares of the tragedy and had become increasingly tired and nervous. He avoided engaging in any activity or conversation in juvenile hall. His appearance was disheveled, his speech slowed, and his attitude signaled defeat. Thomas stated that he didn't care what punishment he received and expected a severe or even capital sentence.

Thomas was diagnosed as suffering from a major depression and PTSD, and psychiatric hospitalization with suicide precautions was recommended. Later reconstruction in psychotherapy indicated that Thomas had shot his sister without intending her to die (*California v. Thomas C* 1986).

Foodman and Estrada (1977) concur that these adolescents experience predominantly guilt and depression complicated by the traumatic symptoms of anxiety, nightmares, and social avoidance. The parents of adolescents who accidentally kill are also plagued by feelings of fear, sadness, and insecurity over their parental ability. A maladaptive parental response will reciprocally reinforce the adolescent's symptomatology and point to the need for early family intervention.

Long-Term Effects

The course of PTSD in adults has been described as demonstrating a phasic variation in predominant symptom type, as an intrusive cluster of re-experiencing, arousal, and nightmares alternates with the numbing responses of denial and ego constriction (Horowitz 1986). It has been further proposed that the pattern of symptoms in Vietnam veterans may also reflect the nature of the trauma, such that witnessing abusive violence is correlated with the re-experiencing phenomena, whereas participating in abusive violence may be significantly related to numbing (Laufer et al. 1985). After several months, chronicity of PTSD may be heralded by an overall diminution in anxiety in the face of increasing social and occupational dysfunction and depression consistent with the sick role.

The natural history of PTSD in adolescents has not been fully elucidated, but evidence is accumulating that its impact on the developing organism can be substantial (Eth 1987). Certainly the experience of catastrophic stress, such as concentration camp confinement, has been shown to have devastating effects on personality formation (Koenig 1964). Lenore Terr's (1983a) study of the Chowchilla school bus kidnapping documented that the early traumatic syndrome persisted over the course of several years. These enduring symptoms included fears, disturbing dreams, behavioral and psychophysiological reenactments, and personality alterations. In addition, Terr noted that in some youngsters there was a delayed onset or progression of symptoms. These typically post-traumatic features were generally unknown to a community control population (Terr 1983b).

Another line of evidence suggests that the capacity for self-control of the young witness of violence may become severely impaired. Examining the most destructive juvenile delinquents in a state detention center, Lewis (1983) found that 78 percent of these adolescents had observed extraordinary violence in their own homes. Ten years after serving in the armed forces as adolescents in Vietnam, a group of Veterans Administration patients were interviewed. These young adults exhibited chronic symptoms of PTSD compounded by drug abuse, rage, and despair. Their profound disillusionment and moral stagnation raised the suspicion that they were languishing in a state of perpetual, pathological adolescence (Jackson 1982).

Case Example

Juan O. is a 15-year-old Hispanic who was admitted to an adolescent day treatment program for persistent dysfunctional behavior. Juan has been suspended from a succession of schools for threatening teachers and fighting with peers. He was finally expelled after being found with a weapon in class. Juan had not had previous psychiatric evaluation or treatment.

About three years earlier Juan witnessed his father's murder in a savage, unprovoked stabbing by a stranger on a street in Mexico. The assailant was never captured. Afterwards Juan's mother moved to California, leaving him in the care of his maternal grandmother. When Juan was reunited with his mother in Los Angeles two years later, he was shocked and dismayed to learn that she had since remarried and given birth. Juan had retained a strong allegiance to his natural father and argued incessantly with his new stepfather.

On psychiatric examination Juan was a small, chubby, bilingual adolescent. He demonstrated conspicuous angry, anxious, and sad affects, but he denied vegetative and ideational signs of depression. Juan evidenced a suspicious, aggressive stance designed primarily to locate and destroy his father's killer. A source of pleasure for Juan was elaborate, heroic revenge fantasies. Juan's provocative hypervigilance had become entrenched despite attempts by family and teachers to spare him the resulting conflicts. Juan received the diagnosis of conduct disorder and PTSD.

Legal Issues

Adolescent witnesses to homicide routinely become involved with the criminal justice system (Pynoos and Eth 1984). The stresses associated with these encounters can cause distress, exacerbate traumatic symptoms, and complicate treatment. The adolescent witness's first contact is with the police, who are the agents responsible for the prompt investigation and arrest of the suspect. In their effort to collect evidence, the police may be insensitive to the plight of a distraught young witness. For instance, the homicide detectives may sequester the adolescent alone in a foreboding police station while awaiting interrogation. The combination of anxiety, isolation, and fatigue erodes the adolescent's ability to respond effectively to questioning. However, a frightened youngster may feel considerably reassured by the protective presence of uniformed officers conducting their investigation. The highly structured police interview is intended to elicit information about the homicide, and its format is often not modified according to the age or emotional condition of the young witness. The detective usually begins by eliciting identifying data from the adolescent and then focuses on the chronological details of the crime, as a rule without pausing to offer understanding or support. Detectives must always be alert to the possibility that a witness may actually have been the perpetrator. This technique differs markedly from the therapeutic interview already described.

The police investigation may lead to the apprehension of a suspect. Depending on the suspect's age, the subsequent proceedings will be conducted either in the juvenile justice system or in the criminal courts. Prior to the actual trial, evidence may need to be presented to a grand jury or at a preliminary hearing. The eyewitness account of the adolescent may represent the foundation of the district attorney's case. Fortunately, the vast majority of adolescents will be found competent to testify, even if asked to demonstrate their cognitive abilities on *voir dire* examination. However, their credibility as witnesses will be a function of whether the jury will trust an adolescent. Many people feel that compared with adults, youngsters have inferior memories and are more suggestible. Recent research has produced results that conflict with this generalization and underscore the complexity of memory for children and adults alike (Goodman 1984). There is no evidence that adolescents are less honest, less able to recall, or are more prone to make false accusations than adults. A goal of cross-examination for all witnesses is to establish the extent to which the independent memory of a crime has been distorted by time or influenced by authority figures. Jury selection by the prosecution and instruction by the judge are critical factors in ensuring that the adolescent's testimony is appreciated for its full weight as evidence.

While testifying in court, the witness is placed directly facing the defendant and spectators. Adolescents know they are being closely scrutinized by a killer as they describe the details of the homicide. Although there are court officials in attendance, the adolescent may feel in serious danger. The reality of their peril should not be minimized. In 1979, 122 youth gangs were responsible for 391 homicides in Los Angeles. According to police sergeant Ben Lovato: "They [gang members] know they can literally get away with murder. The police and the courts cannot protect victims and witnesses. It's almost impossible to get anyone to testify against a gang member; something will happen to people who do—or to their family or their home. So the gang members are not afraid" (Reeves 1981, p. 138). Of course without criminal repercussions the carnage will escalate, involving increasing numbers of killers, victims, and witnesses. Under these circumstances, as is seen in certain inner city areas, an explosive chain reaction occurs. "When society itself is in a state of turmoil, unrest, and danger, the adolescent may then feel impelled toward acts of violence against others or against himself or herself" (Lewis 1982, p. 278).

Case Example

Jane J., 12 years old, was admitted to an adolescent psychiatric ward on the day she was cross-examined in a murder trial. One day before, she had qualified as a witness and had performed competently during direct examination. However, that evening she began to exhibit bizarre behavior and was convinced that her home was under electronic surveillance. She was not accompanied to the court by her mother for the second day of her testimony. The judge excused her as a witness after she appeared confused and disoriented during cross-examination.

Eight months prior to the trial she had disclosed to the police that she had witnessed the shooting of a neighbor by a member of a local gang. She began to fear retaliation from the assailant and his gang shortly after speaking with the police. Her mother, who was also afraid, arranged for her to attend a new school in order to avoid gang members. After the transfer, Jane became disrespectful toward teachers and aggressive with peers for the first time in her school career. She was suspended and transferred four times for classroom fighting during the ensuing eight months.

Jane's mother was opposed to her daughter's court appearance and pressured her to deny that she had witnessed the murder. Convinced that she and her daughter would be jailed if she ignored the subpoena, Mrs. J. finally allowed her daughter to testify. Jane described how she sat facing the defendant and could recall no preparation by the district attorney to familiarize her with the courtroom setting or with the likely content of the cross-examination. Furthermore, she felt alone because of her mother's absence from the courtroom during her second day of testimony.

On admission to the ward Jane believed that her mother was an imposter; she complained of hearing accusatory voices saying, "She didn't even know"; and she was combative when staff members approached her. Physical examination and laboratory studies including drug screen disclosed no abnormalities. There was no family history of psychiatric contact. Inpatient treatment of atypical psychosis and PTSD consisted of neuroleptic medication, psychotherapy, and milieu therapy. Complete remission of psychotic symptoms occurred in six weeks, and at one year follow-up Jane was functioning well at school and was participating in neighborhood activities.

Treatment Issues

During the last 20 years, specific forms of psychotherapy and many promising pharmacological agents have been developed to treat PTSD (Ettedgui and Bridges 1985). Yet the scientific literature for the most part still consists of case reports and un-controlled studies, and very little has been written exclusively about adolescents. Integration of the available material points to a biopsychosocial approach to the traumatized adolescent who has witnessed homicide (Eth et al., in press).

In the biological arena several different classes of psycho-tropic drugs are commonly used to ameliorate the symptoms of PTSD. Benzodiazepines may be prescribed for the short-term relief of anxiety and insomnia in the aftermath of vio-lence. However, the potential of these agents for abuse and dependency is considerable. Both tricyclic and monoamine ox-idase inhibitor antidepressants have been shown to help con-trol the severe symptoms of startle reactions, nightmares, flashbacks, and depression. The antidepressants may require several weeks of administration before substantial improve-ment is noted, and adolescents may complain of the apprecia-ble side effects. Propranolol, lithium, and carbamazepine have all been reported to be efficacious in a small number of experi-mental trials.

Psychological treatments for PTSD abound, ranging from traditional psychoanalytic psychotherapy to behavior modifi-cation and group therapy. Each technique has its own adher-ents and reported successes. If begun soon after the traumatic event, psychodynamic psychotherapy can be conducted in a brief, focal mode allowing for the prompt reduction in stress and the prevention of chronic symptomatology. Therapy de-pends on the establishment of a working alliance fostering open and honest communication—not always an easy task with adolescents. The patient is encouraged to explore the trau-matic event and its aftermath in detail in every session. With each reappraisal the patient should feel in greater control of the associated dysphoric thoughts that correspond with subtle changes in his or her account and an evolution in the quality of his or her dreams from stereotypic nightmares to less intense expression of conflict. The course of psychotherapy is not al-ways smooth, especially as repressed memories are reactivated or as life stresses mount. For many adolescents, coexisting psychopathology including substance abuse also must be confronted. However, by focusing on the trauma-induced crisis, the patient should gain some sense of mastery and as a consequence an expanded array of coping skills.

When the adolescent has enjoyed a meaningful relationship with the homicide victim, grief issues must be managed as well. The treatment should first attend to the more conspicuous elements of psychic trauma. The painful memories of the homicide are intrusive and ego-dystonic and are responsive to early exploration. Following alleviation of the traumatic anxiety, the adolescent will be better able to mourn unencumbered by contamination with traumatic issues. Adolescents who had previously shown no signs of bereavement may then openly grieve in session and be amenable to the comfort and support of the therapist.

The social domain of treatment may assume particular importance for the adolescent when the homicide has disrupted major environmental supports and requires social agency assistance. Another component of sociotherapy is the availability of peer support in the form of self-help groups and organizations. Such activities can help reverse the isolation and estrangement of traumatization and promote removal of social stigma. The availability of special programs, such as the State of California Victim-Witness Assistance Network, may also prove beneficial. The biological, psychological, and social dimensions of therapy for the traumatized adolescent witness to homicide are complementary. A comprehensive treatment plan would naturally encompass those elements appropriate for that particular patient. Although PTSD is a potentially severe affliction; with prompt intervention the prognosis is usually favorable.

Conclusion

In all likelihood large numbers of adolescents will continue to be exposed to homicidal violence. Some of these adolescents cope remarkably well with this experience; most, however, do not, and proceed to develop PTSD. The pathological effects of PTSD on learning, behavior, emotions, and personality in this age group are serious, and the long-term prognosis for the untreated condition may be tragic. Active outreach to these adolescent witnesses, who are easily identified in police reports of the crime, presents a unique, challenging opportunity for secondary and tertiary prevention in the mental health field.

References

American Psychiatric Association: Diagnostic and Statistical Manual of Mental Disorders, Third Edition. Washington, DC, American Psychiatric Association, 1980

American Psychiatric Association: Diagnostic and Statistical Manual of Mental Disorders, Third Edition, Revised. Washington, DC, American Psychiatric Association, 1987

Anderson C: Aspects of pathological grief and mourning. Int J Psychoanal 30:48–55, 1949

Arroyo W, Eth S: Children traumatized by Central American warfare, in Post-Traumatic Stress Disorder in Children. Edited by Eth S, Pynoos RS. Washington, DC, American Psychiatric Press, 1985

Bender L: Children and adolescents who have killed. Am J Psychiatry 116:510–513, 1959

Blum R: Contemporary threats to adolescent health in the United States. JAMA 257:3390–3395, 1987

Burgess AW: Family reaction to homicide. Am J Orthopsychiatry 45:391–398, 1975

California v. Thomas C: 228 Cal. Rptr. 430 (Cal. Ct. App.) 1986

Carek DJ, Watson AS: Treatment of a family involved in fratricide. Arch Gen Psychiatry 11:533–542, 1964

Erikson EH: Childhood and Society, 2nd edition. New York, WW Norton, 1963

Eth S: Adolescent separation-individuation and the court. Bull Am Acad Psychiatry Law 11:231–238, 1983

Eth S: Long-term effects of terrorism in children. West J Med 147:73–74, 1987

Eth S, Pynoos RS: Developmental perspective on psychic trauma in childhood, in Trauma and Its Wake. Edited by Figley CR. New York, Brunner/Mazel, 1985a

Eth S, Pynoos RS: Interaction of trauma and grief in childhood, in Post-Traumatic Stress Disorder in Children. Edited by Eth S, Pynoos RS. Washington, DC, American Psychiatric Press, 1985b

Eth S, Silverstein S, Pynoos RS: Mental health consultation to a preschool following the murder of a mother and child. Hosp Community Psychiatry 36:73–76, 1985

Eth S, Baron DA, Pynoos RS: Death notification. Bull Am Acad Psychiatry Law 15:275–281, 1987

Eth S, Randolph ET, Brown JA: Post traumatic stress disorder, in Modern Perspectives in the Psychiatry of the Neuroses. Edited by Howells JG. New York, Brunner/Mazel (in press)

Ettedgui E, Bridges M: Posttraumatic stress disorder. Psychiatric Clin North Am 8:89–103, 1985

Foodman A, Estrada C: Adolescents who commit accidental homicide. J Am Acad Child Psychiatry 16:314–325, 1977

Freud A: Adolescence. Psychoanal Study Child 13:255–278, 1958

Freud A: Ego and the Mechanisms of Defense (1937). New York, International University Press, 1966

Gardner GE: Aggression and violence—enemies of precision learning in children. Am J Psychiatry 128:445–450, 1971

Goodman GS: Children's testimony in historical perspective. J Social Issues 40(2):9–31, 1984

Group for the Advancement of Psychiatry (GAP): Normal Adolescence. New York, Charles Scribner's Sons, 1968

Horowitz MJ: Stress-response syndromes: a review of posttraumatic and adjustment disorders. Hosp Community Psychiatry 37:241–249, 1986

Horowitz MJ, Wilner N, Kaltreider N, et al: Signs and symptoms of posttraumatic stress disorder. Arch Gen Psychiatry 37:85–92, 1980

Jackson HC: Moral nihilism: developmental arrest as a sequela to combat stress. Adolesc Psychiatry 10:228–242, 1982

Koenig WK: Chronic or persisting identity diffusion. Am J Psychiatry 120:1018–1084, 1964

Krystal H: Trauma and affects. Psychoanal Study Child 33:81–116, 1978

Landgarten HB: Clinical Art Therapy. New York, Brunner/Mazel, 1981

Laufer RS, Brett E, Gallops MS: Symptom patterns associated with posttraumatic stress disorder among Vietnam veterans exposed to war trauma. Am J Psychiatry 142:1304–1311, 1985

Lewis DO: Neuropsychiatric vulnerabilities and violent juvenile delinquency. Psychiatr Clin North Am 6:707–714, 1983

Lewis M: Clinical Aspects of Child Development, 2nd edition. Philadelphia, Lea & Febiger, 1982

Lister ED: Forced silence: a neglected dimension of trauma. Am J Psychiatry 139:872–876, 1982

Morbidity and Mortality Weekly Report: Epidemiologic notes and reports—Los Angeles, 1970–1979. JAMA 225:3348–3351, 1986

Oldham DG: Adolescent turmoil: a myth revisited. Adolesc Psychiatry 6:267–280, 1978

Parkes CM, Weiss RS: Recovery from Bereavement. New York, Basic Books, 1983

Petti TA, Wells K: Crisis treatment of a preadolescent who accidentally killed his twin. Am J Psychother 34:434–443, 1980

Pynoos RS, Eth S: The child as witness to homicide. J Social Issues 40(2):87–108, 1984

Pynoos RS, Eth S: Witness to violence: the child interview. J Am Acad Child Psychiatry 25:306–319, 1986

Reeves R: Hispanic community. New Yorker, September 14, 1981

Rutter M: Resilience in the face of adversity: protective factors and resistance to psychiatric disorders. Br J Psychiatry 147:598–611, 1985

Schetky DH: Role models for violence, in Emerging Issues in Child Psychiatry and the Law. Edited by Schetky DH, Benedek EP. New York, Brunner/Mazel, 1985

Terr LC: Chowchilla revisited: the effects of psychic trauma four years after a school-bus kidnapping. Am J Psychiatry 140:1543–1550, 1983a

Terr LC: Life attitudes, dreams, and psychic trauma in a group of normal children. J Am Acad Child Psychiatry 22:221–230, 1983b

Volkan V: Typical findings in pathological grief. Psychiatr Q 44:231–250, 1970

Wohl A, Kaufman B: Silent Screams and Hidden Cries. New York, Brunner/Mazel, 1985

Chapter 5

Clinicolegal Issues for the Forensic Examiner

GREGORY B. LEONG, M.D.

Chapter 5

Clinicolegal Issues for the Forensic Examiner

*H*omicide, the unlawful killing of another, is one of the most heinous crimes that may be perpetrated. When juveniles or minors commit homicide, many psychiatric-legal issues may be involved. Psychiatric or psychological consultation may be needed to assist the juvenile's attorney in the raising of these clinicolegal issues. Less often does the juvenile court judge or the prosecution raise possible relevant psychiatric-legal issues.

The prevalence of psychiatric disorders in adolescents is not known (Kashani et al. 1987). Less is known diagnostically for preadolescent juveniles, although homicides committed by this age group are very rare (Bender and Curran 1940). Moreover, not all adolescents who commit homicide receive psychiatric evaluations (Malmquist 1971). Thus, the subset of those juveniles who commit homicide and who are mentally ill cannot be easily estimated. Many studies have reported varying rates of mental illness among juveniles who commit homicide (Bender 1939; Cornell et al. 1987; Hellsten and Katila 1965; Lewis et al. 1979, 1983; Rosner et al. 1979; Russell 1973; Sendi and Blomgren 1975; Walshe-Brennan 1977). Definitive conclusions are difficult to draw from these studies. However, they do suggest that although the majority of juveniles who commit homicide are not severely mentally ill, the raising of psychiatric issues in the defense of the juvenile charged with homicide would not be uncommon.

Upon involvement in a juvenile's legal proceedings, the forensic examiner performs a clinical evaluation of the minor. Beyond the clinical assessment of the minor, an awareness of the local legal standards involved in the case is needed. This is

117

mandatory to the formulation of relevant expert opinions, because substantial legal differences may exist among the various jurisdictions. After gathering of clinical data, the reasoning behind the clinician's opinions is crucial to the forensic consultative process (Pollack et al. 1982a, 1982b). Without sound and relevant reasoning, the forensic examiner's clinical opinions may have little value for the courts.

Psychiatric-legal issues that are raised for juveniles include those in common with adult defendants and those unique to juveniles. Many of these issues involve competency. Competency is the capacity to understand the nature of the act to be performed and its consequences. Adult psychiatric-legal issues include competency to waive Miranda rights, competency to stand trial, the insanity defense, and capital case issues. The competency to waive Miranda rights is a more cogent issue for juveniles than for adult defendants. On the other hand, the competency to stand trial, the insanity defense, and capital case issues play a less important role in the juvenile justice system than in the adult criminal system. Psychiatric-legal issues unique to juveniles include juvenile fitness and the infancy defense. These, along with competency to waive Miranda rights, are the mainstay of psychiatric-legal defenses that may be raised for juveniles. These three psychiatric-legal issues are largely determined by the minor's level of maturity and attainment of developmental capacities that are assumed to have been reached by adults.

Upon reaching certain chronological ages, certain mental abilities are assumed to have been developed. Instead of chronological age, the actual developmental attainment of certain cognitive capacities has been suggested as the primary focus in the assessment of various competencies in juveniles (Billick 1986). Oftentimes other biopsychosocial parameters need to be evaluated in order to perform adequate forensic assessment of the juvenile offender. Examples of other parameters include the juvenile's intelligence, school performance, prior judicial experience, and, of course, the presence of mental illness.

Competency to Waive Miranda Rights

The Gault case (*In re Gault* 1967) extended the constitutional rights of juveniles to include many rights afforded to adults, such as Miranda rights. The landmark Miranda case (*Miranda v. Arizona* 1966) provides that a defendant may waive his rights (the right to have an attorney present, the right against self-incrimination, and so forth) so long as the waiver is made voluntarily, knowingly, and intelligently. Additional case law in nonfederal jurisdictions has extended the Miranda ruling for juveniles. For example, the determination of whether or not a minor has knowingly and intelligently waived his rights depends on the minor's age, degree of intelligence, his familiarization with the law or legal proceedings, and the method and duration of the interrogation and similar factors; that is, the waiver depends on the totality of the circumstances, with each case being decided on its own facts (*In re Linda D* 1978).

Studies have cast doubt on juveniles' ability to competently waive their Miranda rights and have suggested that juveniles are less likely than adults to competently waive their Miranda rights (Ferguson and Douglas 1970; Grisso 1981). In the evaluation of minors for competency to waive Miranda rights, the forensic clinician needs to consider all biopsychosocial factors. These include the minor's age, intelligence, cognitive development, school achievement, prior judicial experience, and the presence of mental illness. In arriving at a forensic opinion, cognitive development is likely to be given the most consideration.

Judicial opinion varies as to when a minor is competent to waive his rights, as illustrated in the case of Patrick W. (*In re Patrick W* 1980):

> Thirteen-year-old Patrick W. allegedly shot and killed his police officer stepfather and was arrested on the following day. Patrick was interviewed by sheriff's detectives at 10 p.m., three and one-half hours after his arrest. After being advised of his

Miranda rights, he admitted committing the homicide. The trial court sustained the petition for murder.

The appellate court reversed the trial court's decision on the basis that Patrick was not given the opportunity to talk to his available grandparents prior to his confession. However, of perhaps greater interest were the conflicting opinions given by two of the three appellate court justices. One justice opined that any minor 13 years old or younger is incapable of intelligently and knowingly waiving his Miranda rights. The other judge believed that the transcript of the Miranda waiver in this case demonstrated an intelligent, fairly sophisticated boy of 13 who had given a competent waiver.

The case of Patrick W. illustrates the judicial confusion over what constitutes a competent waiver of Miranda rights. Even though a forensic clinician was not involved in this case, it suggests a need for sound reasoning supported by adequate clinical data when giving an expert opinion regarding this competency.

The following case of Roderick P. (*In re Roderick P* 1980) illustrates the contribution of the psychiatric evaluation in the issue of competency to waive Miranda rights:

Roderick P. was a 14-year-old mentally retarded male of slight build, weighing less than 100 pounds and standing between four and five feet tall. After 9 a.m., a man arrived home from work and found his wife's dead body lying on their living room floor. She was stabbed 19 times, about 8 to 12 hours before her husband's discovery of the body. A teenage neighbor of the dead woman told the police that Roderick was one of the possible perpetrators.

Fifteen hours later, at about 12:15 a.m. of the following day, the police arrived at Roderick's home. He was awakened and read his rights, recited rapidly by the police officer from memory. Roderick's father did not understand them, yet Roderick nodded that he had. When talking to the police officers, Roderick rocked back and forth with his finger in his mouth.

Upon forensic assessment of Roderick, the examining psychiatrist gave a diagnosis of mental retardation. At the court proceedings, the psychiatrist testified that Roderick was mentally retarded, became confused easily, and was passive and susceptible to suggestion. The psychiatrist gave several examples of Roderick's level of intellectual functioning. Roderick was unable to do the following: name the months of the year, state his father's occupation, spell his parents' or sisters' names, or give his sisters' ages. Given his low level of intellectual functioning, Roderick was not likely to have understood more complex questions, including the questions involved in the waiver of Miranda rights. Nevertheless, Roderick would answer questions in a way he believed the interrogator wished to hear in order to avoid conflict with the interviewer.

The psychiatric testimony was unrefuted and unchallenged by the prosecution. Nonetheless, Roderick was found to have committed manslaughter, declared a ward of the court, and sent to a juvenile camp.

On appeal, the California Supreme Court reversed the decision based on two errors. One error was that Roderick's alleged Miranda rights waiver was ineffectual, in light of (clinical) evidence indicating his lack of comprehension of the rights involved in the waiver. The other error was the lack of substantial evidence to support the finding that he had committed the homicide.

Even though the focus of the psychiatric testimony was on Roderick's level of intelligence and cognitive development, other psychological factors played a significant role in explaining Roderick's incompetency to waive Miranda rights. Roderick's passivity, susceptibility to suggestion, and wish to avoid confrontation limited his ability to acknowledge his lack of understanding of his Miranda rights. By answering mechanically in the affirmative, Roderick gave an ineffectual Miranda waiver.

A juvenile's competency to waive Miranda rights is a controversial issue. Not only is the clinical research (Ferguson and Douglas 1970; Grisso 1983) equivocal, judicial opinion also differs as to when juveniles are competent to waive their Miranda rights (*In re Patrick W* 1980). The forensic expert is advised to be as familiar as possible with local standards and case law, so that he or she can evaluate the most relevant and decisive psychological factors for the court.

Juvenile Fitness or Juvenile Waiver into Adult Court

In juvenile court, a separate hearing is conducted if the issue of juvenile fitness or waiver of the juvenile into adult court is raised. When the juvenile is found to be unfit or not appropriate for the juvenile justice system, his or her right to be tried as a juvenile is waived and the case is transferred to the adult criminal court system. Trial by the adult court places the youth at risk for much more severe legal consequences, including life imprisonment and, in some states, the death penalty (Benedek et al. 1987; see also Chapter 7).

Substantial variability exists by jurisdiction for the rules governing juvenile waiver into adult court (Benedek 1985; see also Chapter 8). Juvenile fitness criteria vary as to the minimum age at which a juvenile's case can be waived into adult court and the type of charges that invoke the waiver. Certain offenses automatically waive the juvenile into adult court, unless the defense demonstrates that the minor is fit or appropriate for juvenile court. Guidelines for the waiver of the juvenile into adult court are derived from the Kent case (*Kent v. United States* 1966). The five guidelines include: 1) the prior record and character of the child, his physical and mental maturity, and his patterns of living; 2) the seriousness of the offense; 3) whether the child may be beyond rehabilitation under the regular statutory juvenile procedures; 4) the suitability of programs and facilities available to the juvenile courts for the child; and 5) whether the best interest of public welfare and protection of public security generally requires that a juvenile stand trial as an adult offender (Benedek 1985).

The attorney for the juvenile charged with homicide makes every effort to keep his or her client's case within the juvenile court system. This usually necessitates a forensic clinician's opinion to refute the prosecution's assertion that the juvenile is unfit for the juvenile justice system. When performing a psychiatric consultation for juvenile fitness, the areas of interest in such a consultation include the events of the alleged crime as seen from the juvenile's perspective, the youngster's personal history, family history, school history, social relationships, history of drug and alcohol abuse, prior criminal history, prior mental health treatment, medical treatment, and a mental status examination (Benedek 1985). Unlike the assessment of other clinicolegal issues raised involving competencies, the issue of juvenile fitness requires understanding of the exact legal standard used in the jurisdiction in question in order to render an opinion. This standard is based more upon the local jurisdiction's legal criteria and has less dependence upon the attainment of certain developmental capacities as in the competency to waive Miranda rights, competency to stand trial, and the infancy defense. So long as the local jurisdiction adheres to the federal guidelines (*Kent v. United States* 1966), it may establish its own individualized juvenile fitness criteria. For juveniles charged with homicide, the psychiatric-legal issues of competency to stand trial and negation of criminal responsibility do not play a role in the vast majority of cases, whereas the most important forensic issue in these cases appears to be the juvenile fitness decision (Benedek et al. 1987).

The following case illustrates the forensic clinician's assessment of juvenile fitness (*In re Thomas C* 1986):

Thomas C., a clinically depressed 16-year-old, shot and killed his 14-year-old sister Jody at her request. About a week or two before the homicide, Thomas and Jody, who were very close, ran away together into the hills near their home. After their return, their father took away their keys to the main house. Thomas and Jody were both placed in the bedroom over the detached garage, which previously had been solely Jody's room. They were denied access to the main house, unless their father, stepmother, or stepbrother was present. Thomas's father also took away Thomas's driver's permit as punishment.

On the day prior to the killing, Thomas, Jody, and their father went to the police station for a postrunaway follow-up interview. According to the interviewing detective, Thomas was quiet and withdrawn and appeared depressed. The detective thought Jody also appeared to be depressed. She told the detective she was despondent about having no close friends.

The next day, Thomas burglarized the family home to get

several items, including a .38-caliber revolver, his .22-caliber rifle, his driver's license, a credit card, cash, and two suitcases, because he had decided to run away from home. He took two suitcases to the bedroom over the garage he then shared with Jody, packed his clothes, and lay in the bedroom the entire afternoon. Thomas thought about his immediate plans, including running away to Colorado to visit a girlfriend or perhaps killing himself. When Jody came home, they went for a snack in the family home and then returned to their bedroom. They sat on the bed and began to talk. According to Thomas, she apparently was very despondent and asked him to help her commit suicide. She picked up the handgun from the bed, asked if it was loaded, and indicated she wanted him to kill her. She stood up, went over to the stereo to turn it up, and then walked over to a corner of the room.

Thomas then picked up the handgun and walked over to her. He told her he did not want to do it, but she again reassured him that this was what she wanted. At this time, he directed the weapon at the back of her neck or head area. She told him, "I will count to three and then you shoot." At the count of three, he started to pull the trigger and was very surprised afterwards that he did it. He claimed that he "barely pulled the trigger and was hoping it wouldn't work." Afterwards, there was blood everywhere and he tried to talk to her.

Thomas then wrapped her in a blanket and buried her in the yard. When his parents came home, he appeared upset, claiming someone had burglarized the house. He told his parents that Jody had gone out to visit with friends. His father filed a runaway report for Jody the next day after she failed to attend school. Three days after the shooting, his stepmother found Jody's body under a mound of dirt in the backyard.

Thomas was charged with murder. Five weeks after the shooting, a local child psychiatrist diagnosed Thomas as having major depression with melancholia and recommended psychiatric hospitalization. Because of his age and the type of offense committed, under California law (section 707, California Welfare and Institutions Code) Thomas was assumed to be unfit for the juvenile justice system, unless his attorney could prove otherwise. A forensic child psychiatrist was appointed by the court to assist Thomas's attorney in evaluating whether Thomas was fit for juvenile court and to assess his mental state at the time of the alleged homicide.

The forensic psychiatrist found that Thomas had a long history of episodic depressions. One year prior to the homicide, a psychiatrist prescribed antidepressant medication for Thomas. There was a positive family history for depression, including two probable suicide attempts by Jody. Thomas previously had attempted suicide by overdose at age 14. Also, Jody allegedly tried to help Thomas hang himself. Thomas's upbringing was stressful and chaotic. His biological mother physically abused him. He and Jody were constantly shuttled back and forth between their father and mother during the custody dispute that followed the divorce.

In assessing whether Thomas met the juvenile fitness criteria, the psychiatrist needed to consider the following: 1) the degree of criminal sophistication exhibited by the minor; 2) whether the minor could be rehabilitated prior to the expiration of the juvenile court's jurisdiction; 3) the minor's previous delinquent history; 4) success of previous attempts by the juvenile court to rehabilitate the minor; and 5) the circumstances and gravity of the alleged offense (section 707, California Welfare and Institutions Code). In addition, each of the five criteria required consideration of the minor's amenability to care, treatment, and training programs available through the juvenile court.

The forensic psychiatrist addressed each of these five criteria. For the first criterion, he wrote the following: "The minor is not a cunning or sophisticated sociopath. He is a disturbed, very unhappy young man who has never succeeded in any endeavor." For the second criterion, he wrote: "Not yet 17, there would be more than five years remaining under the [California] juvenile court's jurisdiction. Treatment with appropriate dosage of antidepressant medication should make the minor more amenable to rehabilitation and hopefully protect him from decompensation into overt depressive illness and suicidal behavior." Concerning the third criterion, he wrote: "Prior offenses included joyriding, runaway, and burglary of items from his parent's home. These were consistent with his chronic interpersonal problems and depression." Concerning the fourth criterion, he wrote: "Probation-ordered counseling in Arizona (for the joyriding charge when he went to visit his biological mother) was short-lived and drug therapy apparently was not successful in establishing a therapeutic blood level of anti-depressant. Probation camp and California Youth Authority placement have never been utilized." Finally, in addressing the fifth criterion, he opined that "the tragic death of Jody appeared to have been a misguided mercy killing motivated by the minor's strong suicidal identification with his sister. His own biological state of depression impaired his ability to resist Jody's desperate plea that he put her out of her misery. These mitigating factors, the absence of an alternative exploitative motive for the homicide, the treatability [of] depressive illness, and the minor's recent adoption of a fundamentalist Christianity are favorable indicators for his amenability for rehabilitation."

In order for the minor to qualify for juvenile fitness, the court has to accept the forensic clinician's opinions for each of the five criteria. In Thomas's case, the court agreed with the clinical opinions in all five criteria. Thus, Thomas was found fit for juvenile court. Clearly, the psychiatrist's clinical expertise in assessing and diagnosing Thomas's mental condition was a necessary, but not sufficient, component of his role as expert witness. The forensic examiner must be able to apply clinical findings to the specific legal criteria employed by the court and do so in a clear and convincing manner.

Competency to Stand Trial

Competency to stand trial is a cornerstone of Anglo-American trial procedure. The current legal standard for the determination of competency to stand trial is governed by the Dusky case (*Dusky v. United States* 1960). Competency to stand trial consists of two criteria, both of which must be satisfied for an individual to be competent. One criterion involves whether an accused individual has a rational as well as factual understanding of the proceedings. The other criterion involves whether the accused individual has the present ability to cooperate with his or her attorney with a reasonable degree of rational understanding.

The clinical evaluation for competency to stand trial in adults has been studied (McGarry et al. 1973) and may serve as a model for assessing competency of minors to stand trial. As with evaluations for competency to waive Miranda rights, assessments of juveniles for competency to stand trial must consider both the youth's current mental status and degree of cognitive development. Particular concerns for assessing competency to stand trial in juveniles have been raised (Grisso et al. 1987). As with adults, each minor's case needs to be individually evaluated by consideration of all relevant biopsychosocial parameters. For juveniles, these include age, intelligence, school achievement, prior court experience, the juvenile's demeanor in contacts with counsel, and presence of mental illness (Grisso et al. 1987). These parameters are then evaluated for their effect on the juvenile's understanding of the following: courtroom procedure and personnel, the allegations involved, possible outcomes of the court proceedings, and matters essential to rational cooperation with counsel.

The following case example involves a mentally retarded juvenile charged with first degree murder:

A 15-year-old mentally retarded juvenile (verbal IQ of 55, performance IQ of 77, and full scale IQ of 64, Wechsler Intelligence Scale for Children-Revised) was charged with first degree murder when he stabbed a 35-year-old man to death during a robbery attempt. The minor gave a fantastic version of the alleged offense, stating that he was merely trying to sell the victim a watch when he was attacked by the victim and the victim's friend. The minor added that a passerby fired gunshots at him when he fled the scene. The forensic examiner believed that the minor's version of the offense was an attempt to avoid blame. However, his low level of intellectual functioning contributed to a less than credible version. He was able to demonstrate an understanding of the legal proceedings and the reason he was on trial. He also had past experience with the juvenile court system. Additionally, there was no discernible evidence of a major mental disorder that prevented him from rationally cooperating with his attorney. He was believed to be competent to stand trial despite his mental retardation.

As in adults, determination of juvenile offenders to be incompetent to stand trial is often associated with a current psychotic disorder or severe mental retardation. Since psychotic disorders for the most part do not appear until late adolescence, it would be unlikely for most juvenile offenders to be found incompetent to stand trial. For example, in a series of 50 juveniles charged with homicide who were evaluated at the Center for Forensic Psychiatry in Michigan, only three (6 percent) were recommended by the clinician, and later adjudicated by the court, to be incompetent to stand trial. This sample included only those juveniles referred to the Center for Forensic Psychiatry, with many other juveniles charged with homicide processed directly by the court system (Benedek et al. 1987; see also Chapter 7).

Nonfederal case law exists (*James H v. Superior Court* 1978) that provides juveniles with a right to a hearing to determine their competency to stand trial if a doubt is raised. Nevertheless, many juvenile courts are reluctant to render an incompetency determination. Juvenile courts sometimes fear losing their "control" over the minor's case with an incompetency finding. In such cases, juveniles are relegated to the mental health system, which essentially means the state hospital system. In some jurisdictions, it is generally believed that the psychiatric treatment that is provided in the juvenile justice system is superior to that of the state hospital system, so the juvenile court makes every attempt to keep even a psychiatrically disturbed minor within the juvenile justice system.

When the court disagrees with a forensic clinician's opinion regarding incompetency to stand trial, the forensic evaluation's clinical findings may still be relevant to the minor's case. In the dispositional phase of the trial, many courts would consider evidence of mental illness from a competency report.

Infancy Defense

The infancy defense refers to the concept that underaged individuals are not criminally responsible for their acts. Its roots are from English common law (Platt and Diamond 1966). Under age 7, a juvenile was legally incapable of committing a crime. Between ages 7 and 12, and later between ages 7 and 14, English common law allowed for a guilty finding and even capital punishment. In the United States, between 1806 and 1882, there were 14 recorded cases where the infancy defense was raised for juveniles between the ages of 7 and 14, with 8 of the 14 cases involving a charge of homicide (Platt and Diamond 1966). However, forensic clinicians were not involved in these cases. For example, the jury decided whether an 11-year-old boy qualified for the infancy defense solely on the basis of lay testimony from his neighbors regarding his character and intelligence (*Godfrey v. State* 1858).

Current legal standards for the infancy defense remain similar to the original English common law. Case law may modify the local standard for the infancy defense. In California, minors under the age of 14 are incapable of committing a crime (*People v. Olsen* 1984), unless there is "clear proof" they knew its wrongfulness. In New York, a child under 7 is conclusively presumed incapable of committing a crime and a child between 7 and 14 is rebuttably presumed to lack criminal capacity (*Matter of Andrew M* 1977). Moreover, the nature of the crime alone is not enough to negate the infancy defense, and the juvenile court must consider the child's age, experience, and understanding to determine criminal responsibility (*In re Gladys R* 1971).

In making an assessment involving the infancy defense, the forensic clinician needs to explore a number of factors before offering an expert opinion. These factors may include the minor's intelligence, cognitive development, prior legal experience, moral development, and presence of mental illness. The impact of these factors upon the minor's awareness of wrong-

129

fulness of the alleged act can then be addressed in the forensic clinician's assessment.

The following case illustrates the use of the infancy defense in a charged homicide (*In re Michael B* 1983):

> Nine-year-old Michael B. and 14-year-old John C. were playing together. While riding their bikes, they went to Marty's home where Marty was shooting a BB gun. Michael was permitted to shoot the BB gun, but when he pointed it at John, he was told by Marty not to do so. Michael and John then shot Marty's BB gun.
>
> They left Marty's house and went to Michael's house. Michael's father kept a loaded .22-caliber rifle in the closet to "scare off dogs." Although Michael had once shot the rifle, he had never learned about its safety mechanism or gun safety in general. Nevertheless, Michael's father had "mentioned" to Michael that it was unsafe to point a gun at anyone and had warned Michael to stay away from the gun. Michael also was told not to have playmates in the home when his parents were not at home. Nonetheless, Michael got the rifle out of the closet to show John. John walked over and started to play with videogames. Michael asked John to leave because his parents would be home soon. At this point, Michael knew he had violated two of his parents' rules of playing with the gun and having a visitor in the house without proper supervision. Michael then pointed the gun at John to try to get him to leave. The gun went off and the gunshot hit John in the chest, killing him.
>
> After the shooting, Michael was hysterical, frightened, incoherent, and hyperventilating. He was taken to the local medical emergency room and given an injection of a tranquilizer and a prescription for diazepam. Michael then waived his Miranda rights before his interrogation. He was interrogated five times by the police over the next two days.

At the trial a clinical psychologist testified that Michael had average intellectual ability. Further, the psychologist indicated that Michael was capable of understanding the difference between life and death, but not in the same way as an adult; that is, a nine-year-old boy does not understand the permanence of death. The psychologist also opined that even though a nine-year-old can be aware that a gun kills, this does not necessarily mean that when given a gun, a nine-year-old will behave in a prudent manner to see the gun does not kill.

The juvenile court found that Michael had committed involuntary manslaughter. The court of appeals reversed the trial court's ruling. One reason was cogent to the infancy defense. The appeals court ruled that the evidence given did not constitute "clear proof" that at the time of the shooting, Michael understood the wrongfulness of the charged homicide. Based upon the psychologist's opinions regarding Michael's cognitive development and its impact on his understanding of the wrongfulness of the homicide, the court opined that the evidence did not show beyond a reasonable doubt that Michael fully appreciated the consequences of taking a life, or the permanence of death. Another reason for reversal was the prosecution's failure to prove that Michael competently waived his Miranda rights. Clinical opinion was not cited as a basis for this reason.

Despite its similarity to the insanity defense, the infancy defense substantially depends on the lack of attainment of certain developmental capacities. Other psychiatric-legal defenses that are raised in an attempt to negate criminal responsibility assume the attainment of a certain level of developmental competency. In these cases, a certain level of mental illness is needed even to offer an opinion that negates criminal responsibility. In the infancy defense, a showing of developmental immaturity is more commonly asserted (as in the case of Michael B., above) rather than indicating that mental illness created the incapacity to form the mental state necessary to commit the crime.

Other Criminal Responsibility Tests

Given the trend away from rehabilitation and toward retribution within the juvenile justice system, psychiatric-legal defenses that negate criminal responsibility have taken on increasing importance for many mentally ill juveniles charged with homicide. These forensic issues may be crucial for the minor's legal defense, especially for those severely mentally disturbed minors who are found unfit for the juvenile court and waived into adult criminal court for trial. English common law requires a *mens rea* or criminal mental intent for conviction of a crime. Over the years, different insanity standards to negate the *mens rea* have arisen in Anglo-American law. Presently, virtually all jurisdictions utilize the M'Naghten standard (*Regina v. M'Naghten* 1843), American Law Institute (ALI) standard (section 4.01, American Law Institute, Model Penal Code, proposed official draft, 1962), or their variations for the insanity standard. The M'Naghten standard requires that an individual, at the time of commission of the alleged offense, either was unable to understand the nature and quality of the act or was unable to understand its wrongfulness. The ALI standard requires that an individual, at the time of commission of the alleged offense, lacked substantial capacity either to appreciate the criminality (wrongfulness) of the act or to conform his behavior to the requirements of the law. Other jurisdictional differences involve the burden of proof required and who is required to provide that proof (Callahan et al. 1987). Since the Gault decision (*In re Gault* 1967), states are constitutionally required to apply the insanity defense to juvenile proceedings (Popkin and Lippert 1971). However, the issue of criminal responsibility has not figured prominently in the juvenile courts, because traditionally it has been considered a noncriminal system (Harrington and Keary 1980).

Forensic clinicians rarely give an opinion supporting insanity for juveniles charged with homicide (Benedek et al. 1987). A possible reason for the rarity of the insanity defense in juvenile proceedings is that, as with adult defendants who are found not guilty by reason of insanity, juveniles who are believed to qualify for the insanity defense are generally psychotic. As noted earlier, most psychotic disorders only begin to appear in adolescence. Thus, the likelihood of juveniles who commit homicide qualifying for the insanity defense would be rare.

132

In some jurisdictions, if the minor is found not guilty by reason of insanity, the juvenile delinquency petition is dismissed. Unless the minor meets civil commitment criteria, a treatment disposition is not possible (Popkin and Lippert 1971). This is in contrast to the finding of not guilty by reason of insanity for adults, where such a determination generally carries commitment to a psychiatric facility when a mental disorder continues to be active. Thus, after completion of the legal proceedings, the juvenile justice system is reluctant to have a juvenile without a rehabilitative disposition. Moreover, judges and attorneys in the juvenile justice system oftentimes prefer that a mentally ill minor remain with the juvenile justice system to receive psychiatric care, rather than be transferred to the state hospital system. Even if the forensic clinician's opinion supporting legal insanity is not accepted, the forensic report may assist in the dispositional plan for the minor.

Guidelines for evaluating an adolescent for the insanity defense have been suggested (Palombi 1980). These guidelines do not differ from those used in the assessment of insanity for an adult defendant. In assessing the mental state of the juvenile offender at the time of the alleged homicide, all relevant biopsychosocial data need to be gathered. Besides clinical evaluation of the minor, collateral evidence (for example, accounts of eyewitnesses, police reports) regarding the juvenile's mental state at and around the time of the alleged homicide is crucial to the assessment of insanity. Sound reasoning linking the gathered data to the applicable insanity standard is the final step before offering a clinicolegal opinion of insanity.

Besides the insanity defense, other psychiatric-legal defenses are available to juveniles charged with homicide. The variations of diminished capacity, diminished responsibility, or partial insanity negate critical elements of the homicide charge. In all jurisdictions, certain mental states need to be present to convict an individual of murder. In many jurisdictions, mental impairment at the time of the commission of the alleged homicide can negate the ability to premeditate, deliberate, harbor malice aforethought, and/or form the intent to

133

kill. The absence of these mental states may reduce a charge of first degree murder to second degree murder, a charge of second degree murder to voluntary manslaughter, and so forth.

The previously discussed case of Thomas C. (*In re Thomas C* 1986), who killed his sister, illustrates the attempt to reduce the severity of the charged homicide. The defense's basis for the proposed reduction of the charge was the negation of the minor's ability to form the mental states at the time of the alleged homicide that are required for a murder conviction.

The psychiatrist opined that Thomas was not psychotic or delusional at the time of shooting his sister. However, the psychiatrist asserted that Thomas's depression, his suicidal ideation, and the pressure of Jody's demand impaired Thomas's ability to deliberate, premeditate, and harbor malice aforethought. In California, all three mental states are required for a finding of first degree murder, while harboring malice aforethought is required for second degree murder.

The court agreed with the forensic examiner that Thomas's confused mental state precluded the kind of reflective process involved in premeditation and deliberation. However, the court disagreed with the expert opinion that Thomas's mental state prevented him from harboring malice aforethought. The court believed that Thomas did harbor malice aforethought, because he was fully aware that placing a gun to his sister's head and pulling the trigger would cause her death. Since the court opined Thomas did harbor malice aforethought, but did not premeditate and deliberate, the petition was sustained for the lesser charge of second degree murder and not first degree murder. The court of appeals affirmed the original decision.

Psychiatric Participation in Capital Cases

In *Thompson v. Oklahoma*, the United States Supreme Court ruled the death penalty unconstitutional for a defendant who committed a capital crime as a juvenile (*Thompson v. Oklahoma* 1988). However, the Court left open the possibility that state legislatures could explicitly authorize the death penalty for juveniles in the future. Some states forbid capital punishment of juveniles, even when the minor was tried in adult court (*People v. Davis* 1981; *People v. Spears* 1983; Brody 1986). Other states do not forbid the death penalty for juveniles of any age (Brody 1986). The very existence of the death penalty for those who commit homicide while of juvenile age is controversial within the legal community (Anders 1986; Brody 1986). Forensic clinicians may participate in capital cases to give consultation primarily on two issues.

The major issue involving psychiatric participation in capital cases occurs in the sentencing phase of juveniles convicted of homicide. In those states where capital sentencing is allowed for juveniles, psychiatric opinions may be utilized by either the prosecution or defense to bolster their respective arguments for or against the death penalty for the convicted juvenile. Forensic opinions that contain primarily aggravating factors in support of the prosecutorial position do not need to be based on a clinical interview of the defendant, but may be based on responses to hypothetical questions (*Barefoot v. Estelle* 1983). On the other hand, the Supreme Court requires that the judge consider any aspect of a defendant's character or record and any circumstances of the offense that could serve as a basis for a sentence less than death (*Lockett v. Ohio* 1978). The forensic clinician's evaluation may be particularly useful in the assessment of mitigating factors involving psychiatric or psychological issues that could reduce the likelihood that the juvenile receives the death penalty.

The following case illustrates the use of the psychiatric consultant's opinion of mitigating factors in the sentencing phase of a first degree murder conviction (*Eddings v. Oklahoma* 1982):

> Eddings, a 16-year-old, and several younger companions ran away from their Missouri homes. They traveled in a car owned by Eddings's brother and eventually crossed into Oklahoma. Eddings had a shotgun and several rifles, which he had taken from his father, in the car. He was signaled to pull over by an Oklahoma Highway Patrol officer, because the officer had ob-

served Eddings momentarily losing control of his car. Eddings pulled over. As the officer approached the car, Eddings stuck a loaded shotgun out of the window and fired, killing the officer.

Eddings was charged with first degree murder and stood trial as an adult. He was convicted of first degree murder after pleading no contest.

A psychiatric consultation was obtained to assist in the sentencing proceedings. Eddings's parents were divorced when he was five. He lived with his mother until age 14 without rules or supervision. There was suggestion that his mother was an alcoholic and a prostitute. At 14, he was sent to live with his father to control him. He received substantial physical punishment from his father.

At the trial, the psychiatrist testified that Eddings could be rehabilitated by intensive therapy over a 15- to 20-year period. The psychiatrist suggested that, at the time of the murder, Eddings was in his mind shooting his stepfather, a policeman who had married his mother for a brief period when he was seven. The psychiatrist further testified that "given the circumstances and the facts of his life, and the facts of his arrested development, he acted as a seven-year-old seeking revenge and rebellion," and "he did pull the trigger, he did kill someone, but I don't think he knew what he was doing."

The trial court sentenced Eddings to death. On appeal to the Oklahoma Court of Appeals, the sentence was affirmed. On a writ of certiorari, the United States Supreme Court in a five to four decision reversed in part and remanded the case, based on the state trial judge's refusal to consider Eddings's family history and emotional disturbance in mitigation. The legal basis for the decision lay in the violation of the Eighth and Fourteenth Amendments.

Eddings's turbulent family, history of physical abuse by his father, and asserted immaturity offered by the forensic examiner as mitigating factors did not legally or morally negate his responsibility for the homicide. Nevertheless, the judge is required to consider factors of mitigation in the decision to assess the death penalty.

The competency-to-be-executed issue has not yet been raised for juveniles. Presently, it is a rare clinicolegal issue for adults. The competency-to-be-executed issue arises when by reason of a mental illness, a death row inmate is believed to be unable to appreciate the finality of the execution and the reason for the execution. Although the forensic issue is straightforward, the ethical dilemmas raised are highly problematic (Appelbaum 1986; Radelet and Barnard 1986; Salguero 1986). Unless the Supreme Court forbids the death penalty for crimes committed as minors, the competency-to-be-executed issue may arise for a juvenile in the future.

Conclusion

An overview of psychiatric-legal issues applicable to juveniles who commit homicide has been presented. The variety of clinicolegal issues involves the different phases of the legal process beginning with the arrested minor's competency to waive Miranda rights and ending with psychiatric participation in cases of juveniles convicted of homicide who may be given the death penalty. The psychiatric-legal issues of the competency to waive Miranda rights, the infancy defense, and the juvenile fitness issue have particular relevance for juveniles.

Forensic consultations in cases of juveniles who are charged with or who have committed homicide may be a challenging task. Besides having the requisite psychiatric knowledge and skills to do a clinical assessment with a forensic focus, the forensic clinician must know the psychiatric-legal issues involved, and the legal standards in the jurisdiction where the homicide occurred have importance in formulating opinions for the legal system.

This chapter has only briefly highlighted the issues encountered by the forensic clinician consulting on cases involving juveniles charged with homicide. For a more thorough understanding of these forensic issues, additional education is suggested via fellowship training, postgraduate courses in forensic psychiatry and psychology, and/or the study of the clinical forensic literature.

A thorough clinical biopsychosocial data base and sound

reasoning for the offered opinions form the basis for competent forensic consultation in these cases. No matter how scientific the clinical assessment may be and how certain the forensic clinician is of his or her opinions, the clinician remains a consultant to the courts. The juvenile court judge is always the decision maker in the juvenile justice system.

References

Anders JC: Punish the guilty. American Bar Association Journal 72:32–33, 1986

Appelbaum PS: Competence to be executed: another conundrum for mental health professionals. Hosp Community Psychiatry 37:682–684, 1986

Bender L: Children and adolescents who have killed. Am J Psychiatry 116:510–513, 1939

Bender L, Curran FJ: Children and adolescents who kill. Journal of Criminal Psychopathology 1:297–322, 1940

Benedek EP: Waiver of juveniles to adult court, in Emerging Issues in Child Psychiatry and the Law. Edited by Schetky DH, Benedek EP. New York, Brunner/Mazel, 1985

Benedek EP, Cornell DG, Staresina L: Juvenile homicide: a follow-up of forensic outcome. Presented at the 140th Annual Meeting of the American Psychiatric Association, Chicago, IL, May 14, 1987

Billick S: Development competency. Bull Am Acad Psychiatry Law 14:301–309, 1986

Brody RJ: Don't kill the children. American Bar Association Journal 72:32–33, 1986

Callahan L, Mayer C, Steadman HJ: Insanity defense reforms in the United States—post-Hinckley. Mental and Physical Disability Law Reporter 11:54–59, 1987

Cornell DG, Benedek EP, Benedek DM: Characteristics of adolescents charged with homicide: a review of 72 cases. Behavioral Sciences and the Law 5:11–23, 1987

Ferguson B, Douglas AC: A study of juvenile waiver. San Diego Law Review 7:39–54, 1970

Grisso T: Juveniles' Waiver of Rights: Legal and Psychological Competency. New York, Plenum Press, 1981

Grisso T, Miller MO, Sales B: Competency to stand trial in juvenile court. International Journal of Psychiatry and Law 10:1–20, 1987

Harrington MM, Keary AO: The insanity defense in juvenile delinquency proceedings. Bull Am Acad Psychiatry Law 8:272–279, 1980

Hellsten P, Katila O: Murder and other homicide, by children under 15 in Finland. Psychiatr Q Suppl 39:54–74, 1965

Kashani J, Beck NC, Hopper EW, et al: Psychiatric disorders in a community setting of adolescents. Am J Psychiatry 144:584–589, 1987

Lewis DO, Shanok SS, Pincus JH, et al: Violent juvenile delinquents: psychiatric, neurological, psychological and base factors. J Child Psychiatry 18:307–319, 1979

Lewis DO, Shanok SS, Grant M, et al: Homicidally aggressive young children: neuropsychiatric and experiential correlates. Am J Psychiatry 140:148–153, 1983

Malmquist CP: Premonitory signs of homicidal aggression in juveniles. Am J Psychiatry 128:461–465, 1971

McGarry AL, Lipsett PD, Lelos D: Competency to Stand Trial and Mental Illness: Final Report. DHEW publ. no. (HSM) 73-9105. Rockville, MD, National Institute of Mental Health, 1973

Palombi JJ: Competency and criminal responsibility, in Emerging Issues in Child Psychiatry and the Law. Edited by Schetky DH, Benedek EP. New York, Brunner/Mazel, 1980

Platt A, Diamond BL: The origins of the "right and wrong" test of criminal responsibility and its subsequent development in the United States: an historical survey. California Law Review 54:1227–1258, 1966

Pollack S: Principles of forensic psychiatry for reaching psychiatric-legal opinions: introduction, in The Mental Health Professional and the Legal System. Edited by Gross BH, Weinberger LE. San Francisco, Jossey-Bass, 1982a

Pollack S: Principles of forensic psychiatry for reaching psychiatric-legal opinions: application, in The Mental Health Professional and the Legal System. Edited by Gross BH, Weinberger LE. San Francisco, Jossey-Bass, 1982b

Popkin AB, Lippert FJ: Is there a constitutional right to the insanity defense in juvenile court? Journal of Family Law 10:421–442, 1971

Radelet ML, Barnard GW: Ethics and the psychiatric determination of competency to be executed. Bull Am Acad Psychiatry Law 14:37–53, 1986

Rosner R, Wiederlight M, Rosner MBH, et al: Adolescents accused of murder and manslaughter: a five-year descriptive study. Bull Am Acad Psychiatry Law 7:342–351, 1979

Russell DH: Juvenile murderers. International Journal of Offender Therapy and Comparative Criminology 17:235–239, 1973

Salguero RG: Medical ethics and competency to be executed. Yale Law Journal 96:167–186, 1986

Sendi IB, Blomgren PG: A comparative study of predictive criteria in the predisposition of homicidal adolescents. Am J Psychiatry 132:423–427, 1975

Walshe-Brennan KS: A socio-psychological investigation of young murderers. British Journal of Criminology 17:58–63, 1977

Cases Cited

Barefoot v. Estelle, 463 U.S. 880, 1983

Dusky v. United States, 362 U.S. 402, 1960

Eddings v. Oklahoma, 71 L. Ed. 2d 1, 1982

Godfrey v. State, 31 Ala. 323, 1858

In re Gault, 387 U.S. 1, 1967

In re Gladys R, 1 Cal. 3d 855, 1971

In re Linda D, 3 Cal. App. 3d 567, 1978

In re Michael B, 149 Cal. App. 3d, 1973, 1983

In re Patrick W, 84 Cal. App. 3d 520, 1978; vacated *California v. Patrick W*, 61 L. Ed. 2d 870, 1979, on remand 104 Cal.

App. 3d 615, 1980; certiorari denied 66 L. Ed. 2d 824, 1981

In re Roderick P, 7 Cal. 3d 801, 1972

In re Thomas C, 183 Cal. App. 3d 786, 1986

James H v. Superior Court, 77 Cal. App. 3d 169, 1978

Kent v. United States, 383 U.S. 541, 1986

Lockett v. Ohio, 57 L. Ed. 2d 870, 1978

Matter of Andrew M, 398 N.Y.S. 2d 824, 1977

Miranda v. Arizona, 384 U.S. 436, 1966

People v. Davis, 29 Cal. 3d 814, 1981

People v. Olsen, 36 Cal. 3d 638, 1984

People v. Spears, 33 Cal. 3d 279, 1983

Regina v. M'Naghten, 10 Cl. & F. 200, 8 Eng. Rep. 718, 1843

Thompson v. Oklahoma, 56 USLW 4892 (1988)

Competency to Stand Trial and Criminal Responsibility in the Juvenile Court

W. LAWRENCE FITCH, J.D.

Chapter 6

Competency to Stand Trial and Criminal Responsibility in the Juvenile Court

At common law, before the advent of the juvenile court, children who committed crimes were prosecuted in much the same manner as adults. Any defense that an adult could raise, including the insanity defense, the child could raise as well. In addition, younger children were protected by the defense of "infancy."

The infancy defense at common law provided that children under the age of seven years conclusively were presumed to be incapable of committing a crime. Either because they were unable to form criminal intent or because they were unable to make moral judgments of right and wrong, they could not be held criminally responsible for their behavior. Children between the ages of 7 and 14 years were presumed not to be capable of committing a crime, but that presumption was rebuttable. If a child in this age range were charged with a crime, the state would have to prove beyond a reasonable doubt that the child was able to distinguish between "good and evil" if a conviction were to result (*Ford v. State* 1891). Children over the age of 14 years were treated as adults under the common law.

During the nineteenth century a movement was begun to reform the manner in which children who violated the law were handled. The movement was grounded in the belief that "[m]any of these are young people on whom the charge of crime can not be fastened, and whose only fault is, that they have no one on earth to take care of them, and that they are incapable of providing for themselves" (Society for the Prevention of Pauperism 1823). The focus of this movement was on diversion from the criminal courts and treatment as an alternative to punishment.

In 1899, Illinois became the first state to establish a separate juvenile court for dealing with troubled youths. The jurisdiction of the Illinois Juvenile Court was extremely broad, encompassing not only behavior that otherwise would be criminal but other "unhealthy" behavior as well. Moreover, no child was considered too young to be subject to the jurisdiction of the court. By the early 1920s, juvenile courts had been established throughout the country. The central purpose of these courts was rehabilitation. Assessment of guilt and imposition of punishment had no place in the early days of the American juvenile court. The one exception, written into the juvenile court acts of many states, was that juveniles above a certain age who were deemed not suitable for the benevolent intervention of the juvenile court could be "transferred" out of the juvenile court to be tried as adults. Ordinarily, whether or not to transfer the juvenile was a matter within the juvenile court's discretion. In some states, however, juveniles above a certain age who were charged with very serious offenses—notably homicide—were transferred automatically.

With the rise of the juvenile court, the infancy defense and the insanity defense fell out of use. In a system designed to serve rather than punish troubled youths, these defenses were seen as irrelevant, based as they were on questions of moral blameworthiness. Moreover, "[i]f a child did not know that what he did was wrong [a key issue for both the insanity defense and the infancy defense], so much more did he need to be reformed" (Fox 1970, p. 662).

Not only were the juvenile courts more paternal in their philosophy than the adult criminal courts, but the procedures under which they operated were significantly more relaxed as well. The kinds of formal evidentiary rules and other due process protections that characterized American criminal procedure were virtually nonexistent in the early juvenile court. It was believed that if any information could shed light on the problems of a child, that information should be considered, without regard for legal technicality (Weissman 1983). With so little concern for adversarial due process, it did not matter that the child was unable to understand the legal proceedings or mount a defense. Accordingly, questions of the child's competency to stand trial rarely were raised in the juvenile court.

For nearly half a century, the juvenile court in this country took an informal, paternalistic approach to the problems of juvenile delinquency. By the 1960s, however, it had become clear that this approach had failed. Critics cited the "vagaries" of the juvenile court process and the "harsh realities of its institutions" (Walkover 1984, p. 517).

> It has not succeeded significantly in rehabilitating delinquent youths, in reducing or even stemming the tide of juvenile criminality, or in bringing justice or compassion to the child offender. ... [I]n fact the same purposes that characterized the use of the criminal law for adult offenders—retribution, condemnation, and incapacitation—are involved in the disposition of juvenile offenders too. (President's Commission on Law Enforcement and Administration of Justice 1967, p. 8)

In a decision that would have a significant impact on the direction of the juvenile court movement in this country, *In re Gault* (1967), the United States Supreme Court reasoned that, because the juvenile courts had failed to deliver on their promise to use their broad discretionary powers to provide treatment free from punishment, children facing delinquency adjudication in juvenile court constitutionally were entitled to many of the same procedural protections accorded to adult criminal defendants (*In re Gault* 1967). The *Gault* case involved a 15-year-old boy, Gerald Gault, who was adjudicated delinquent by an Arizona juvenile court for "making lewd telephone calls" and was committed to the Arizona State Industrial School until his 21st birthday. At his hearing in juvenile court, Gault was afforded no access to counsel, no opportunity to confront or cross-examine his accuser, and no privilege against self-incrimination. After his hearing, he was afforded no right to appeal to a higher court. The case finally reached the United States Supreme Court on habeas corpus review. Observing that the maximum penalty that Gault could have received had he been 18 years old at the time of the offense was a fine of $5 to $50 or imprisonment in jail for not more than two months, and that, had he been 18, he would have been entitled to "substantial" constitutional and state statutory rights, the Supreme Court in *Gault* chided the juvenile court for its pretensions of paternalism and blasted the juvenile court model as inadequate for the dispensation of justice. "Juvenile court history has again demonstrated that unbridled discretion, however benevolently motivated, is frequently a poor substitute for principle and procedure ..." (*In re Gault* 1967, p. 18). "Under our Constitution, the condition of being a boy does not justify a kangaroo court ... " (*In re Gault* 1967, p. 28). In the end, the court held that juveniles facing delinquency proceedings were entitled to written notice of charges, the right to be represented by counsel, the privilege against self-incrimination, and the right to confront and cross-examine witnesses.

Subsequent Supreme Court decisions have recognized additional due process protections, including the right to have allegations proved beyond a reasonable doubt (*In re Winship* 1970) and the right not to be tried for the same offense twice (*Breed v. Jones* 1975). With this "criminalization" of the juvenile court over the last 20 years, new interest has been shown in questions of juveniles' competency to stand trial and criminal responsibility.

Competency to Stand Trial

The doctrine of competency to stand trial provides that no person shall be subjected to trial on a criminal charge unless he or she has "sufficient present ability to consult with his lawyer with a reasonable degree of rational understanding—and . . . a rational as well as factual understanding of the proceedings against him (*Dusky v. United States* 1960, p. 402). Defendants found incompetent to stand trial ordinarily are admitted automatically to mental health treatment facilities for restoration of competency. If it is determined that the defendant cannot be restored in the "foreseeable future," however, the defendant must be released from such treatment unless he or she agrees to remain as a voluntary patient or is committed pursuant to civil standards and procedures (*Jackson v. Indiana* 1972).

In their original, nonadversarial form, the juvenile courts held no place for consideration of the accused child's competency to stand trial. If the child had no right to be represented by counsel, certainly there was no need that he or she have the ability to consult with counsel with a reasonable degree of rational understanding. Moreover, because disposition in the juvenile court was intended to address the best interests of the child, rather than retributive concerns, no need was seen to protect the child from the consequences of adjudication. Indeed, if the child was so mentally or emotionally disturbed as to be considered incompetent to stand trial, then almost certainly, it seemed, disposition in the juvenile court would entail treatment for that disturbance, the same as if he or she had been found incompetent.

With the recognition since *Gault*, however, that alleged delinquents in fact face a risk of substantial loss of liberty at the hands of the juvenile court and, thus, are entitled to significant due process protection, the question of juveniles' competency to stand trial has been revived. Today, 17 states and the District of Columbia explicitly recognize the right of a juvenile charged with a delinquency offense to be competent to stand trial (Grisso et al. 1987). Many of these states provide the right by statute. Others have recognized the right by court decision. For example, in the case, *In the Interest of Causey,* the Louisiana Supreme Court ruled that fundamental fairness under the due process clause of the Fourteenth Amendment to the United States Constitution required consideration of compe-

149

tency to stand trial for a 16-year-old charged with armed robbery, where the report of a psychologist indicated that the child's intellectual functioning varied "from the upper end of the range of moderate mental retardation with regard to nonverbal intelligence ... to the range of mild mental retardation with regard to verbal intelligence ... " (*In re Causey* 1978, p. 476). "Indeed," the court reasoned, "the right—rooted as it is in traditional notions of fair play, viewed from the early days of the common law as central to a defendant's ability to present his defense, and akin to the right not to be tried *in absentia*—is not only historically fundamental, but also functionally essential, and therefore cannot be outweighed under the *Gault/McKeiver/Winship* test by other, desirable aspects of the juvenile system" (*In re Causey* 1978, p. 476).

Although no court expressly has rejected application of the competency doctrine in the juvenile court, a few states effectively preclude consideration of juveniles' competency by prohibiting mental health evaluations prior to an adjudication of delinquency (Grisso et al. 1987). In these states, an evaluation of the juvenile's mental condition may be conducted only after it is determined that the juvenile committed the offense charged; if at this stage mental health treatment is deemed necessary, the case may be disposed of accordingly.

Certainly it can be argued that if the disposition would be the same whether a determination of incompetency were made or not, such a determination would be superfluous. Other, social disabilities, however, have been recognized to flow from an adjudication of delinquency, such as the stigma of the delinquency label ("only slightly less" stigmatizing than the label, "criminal," observed the Supreme Court in *Gault*) (*In re Gault* 1967, p. 24). Therefore, apart from considerations of disposition, there remains a sound basis for the argument that children must in all fairness be provided a meaningful opportunity to defend against allegations of delinquency.

In most states in which the issue of competency to stand trial is recognized in juvenile court, the standard for determining competency is the same as that applied to adults—the standard articulated in *Dusky*. In the *Causey* case, discussed above, however, the Louisiana Supreme Court alluded to the inherently reduced ability of juveniles to understand legal procedures and cooperate with counsel, suggesting that perhaps the standard for competency in the juvenile court might reasonably be lower than the standard applicable in adult criminal court (*In re Causey* 1978). But the difference at issue here is a matter of degree, not one of quality. Accordingly, the focus of inquiry where the question of competency is raised is the same whether the subject of the inquiry is 7 or 70 years old: is the individual's capacity to understand the proceedings and assist in his or her defense sufficiently well developed to enable the individual to receive a fair trial?

Whether or not someone—an adult or a juvenile—is able to receive a fair trial, of course, is a social value judgment. The clinician may have much to say about the effects of the individual's immaturity or abnormal mental condition on his or her capacity to understand the proceedings and cooperate with counsel, but, ultimately, whether the individual's capacity is so significantly impaired as to require a finding of incompetency is for the court to decide.

The Insanity Defense

The insanity defense has developed in Anglo-American law over several hundred years. Its purpose is to protect against the conviction and punishment of persons who cannot justly be blamed for their behavior. In about half of the states, a criminal defendant may be found not guilty by reason of insanity if at the time of the offense charged, because of a "mental disease or defect," he or she "lacked substantial capacity either to appreciate the wrongfulness of his conduct or to conform his conduct to the requirements of the law" (American Law Institute Model Penal Code 1962). Other tests for legal insanity have been devised in different states, but nearly all require a similar quality of cognitive or volitional impairment induced by serious mental disorder (Favole 1983). In most states, persons acquitted by reason of insanity may be involuntarily committed for psychiatric treatment under a different—and less libertarian—set of standards and procedures than apply to civil commitment. Although controversial, such commitment laws have been approved by the United States Supreme Court (*Jones v. United States* 1983).

A related concern, often confused with the defense of insanity, is the question of *mens rea*. The *mens rea* "doctrine," as currently understood, holds that unless the prosecution establishes that at the time of the offense the defendant acted with the quality of intent, or *mens rea,* that constitutes an element of the offense charged, no conviction may ensue. For example, if the defendant is charged in the shooting death of an acquaintance during a hunting trip, and it is established that the shooting was accidental—that the defendant mistook the victim for a deer—then the defendant cannot be convicted of first degree murder, because the offense of first degree murder requires a *mens rea* of "premeditation" or "purpose"; nor could the defendant be convicted of second degree murder, because this offense requires a *mens rea* of "malice aforethought" or "knowledge." The defendant, however, may be subject to conviction on a charge of voluntary manslaughter, which requires a *mens rea* of "recklessness," or involuntary manslaughter, which requires a *mens rea* of "negligence." If there is no related, less serious offense whose *mens rea* the defendant satisfied, the defendant simply would be acquitted. Ordinarily, defendants acquitted on this basis are not subject to post-acquittal commitment.

Before *Gault,* neither the insanity defense nor the concept of *mens rea* received significant attention in the juvenile courts. The insanity defense in particular was considered simply inapplicable in juvenile court because determinations of blameworthiness and imposition of punishment were not among the court's purposes. However, with the growing recognition in the last 20 years that, in fact, punishment plays a role in the juvenile court, questions of legal insanity have been raised with increasing frequency. Most courts that have considered the issue in recent years have ruled that the insanity defense *should* be available in juvenile court. In approving the defense for a 15-year-old schizophrenic boy charged with the murder of his mother, the Wisconsin Supreme Court asked: "Is it fair to convict of crime when the defendant, though knowing right from wrong, as a result of mental illness or incapacity, is unable to exercise the restraints upon his conduct that would enable him to conform to acceptable standards? It would seen incongruous that this great outpouring of concern should be lavished only upon adults who may be criminals while the children whom we profess to be particular objects of solicitude are bypassed" (*Winburn v. Wisconsin* 1966, p. 184).

Since the Supreme Court's opinion in *Gault,* only two courts have rejected the insanity defense for juveniles, a trial court in New Jersey (in the case of a 15-year-old schizophrenic boy who allegedly killed two young girls) (*In re H.C.* 1969) and the District of Columbia Court of Appeals (in a case involving a mentally ill child, age not given, who was charged with taking indecent liberties with a younger child) (*In re C.W.M.* 1979). In both of these cases, the court's rationale was simple: if rehabilitation, and not punishment, is the purpose of a delinquency adjudication, then a doctrine which has as its sole purpose the prevention of unjust punishment must be irrelevant. The New Jersey court observed that "to hold insanity applicable as a defense to adjudication would handcuff the court, run contrary to the basic theory of juvenile proceedings, and not be in the best interests of the juvenile himself" (*In re H.C.* 1969, p. 328). The D.C. court suggested that if, in fact, the insanity defense served some function essential to fundamental fairness (that is, to treat rather than punish persons whose offensive behavior was not culpable), that same function could be served by procedures mandating consideration of the juvenile's mental disorder and need for treatment at disposition (*In re C.W.M.* 1979). In 1975, the New Jersey decision was overruled by the Superior Court of New Jersey (*In re R.G.W.* 1975), leaving the District of Columbia as the only jurisdiction in which denial of an insanity defense for juveniles explicitly is endorsed. Of course, many states have not yet ruled on the matter.

Administration of the insanity defense traditionally has posed problems in adult criminal cases, and it can be anticipated that many of these problems will be exacerbated in juvenile court. For example, the unreliability of psychiatric opinion, which sometimes provokes a "battle of the experts" in criminal cases, may be heightened in juvenile cases, given the difficulty with which differential diagnosis is made in children (Kolvin 1971). In addition, determining the extent to which mental disorder, as opposed to simple immaturity, was responsible for a child's inability to appreciate the wrongfulness of his or her behavior might prove difficult in some cases.

Procedures for the treatment and release of insanity acquittees also can be expected to raise problems in juvenile cases. Many observers have complained that procedures of the type endorsed by the United States Supreme Court in *Jones v. United States*—procedures that permit insanity acquittees as a group to be subjected to more restrictive treatment conditions than other patients, regardless of their degree of mental disorder or dangerousness—run counter to the central, exculpatory theme of the insanity defense (Stone 1982). If these more restrictive procedures are adopted in juvenile court, where treatment ostensibly is the goal even upon a finding of delinquency, the purpose of the insanity defense—again, to protect against the "punitive" consequences of adjudication—will have been turned on its head.

As a practical matter, of course, it is not likely that the insanity defense often will be raised in juvenile court. To begin with, the kinds of major mental disorders that typically provide the basis for the defense of insanity in adult cases—notably schizophrenia (Warren and Fitch 1987)—may be less frequently diagnosed in juveniles (Kolvin 1971). Furthermore, despite the accepted view that the juvenile court has retributive features, in most states, for most offenses, juvenile court dispositions are likely to be significantly less severe than the kinds of sentences imposed for the same conduct in adult criminal court; thus, juveniles should have even less incentive than adults to pursue this "last ditch" defense. Finally, given the wide discretion of the juvenile court to fashion a disposition that addresses the needs of the juvenile, it is likely that the juvenile who is so disturbed as to qualify for an insanity defense will receive treatment whether or not a finding of insanity is made. Thus, again, this defense should hold little interest for the vast majority of delinquency defendants.

The *mens rea* concept, on the other hand, should hold great appeal for children facing delinquency proceedings, given the dispositional advantages it presents. Very few reported cases, however, have addressed the applicability of this concept in juvenile court. Of those that have, none has rejected the concept and at least one expressly has endorsed it (overturning a juvenile court's adjudication of delinquency for an accidental shooting) (*In re Glassberg* 1956). As McCarthy observes, however, it is a relatively simple matter in many cases for the juvenile court to adhere to the technical requirements of *mens rea* and proceed with adjudication nonetheless (McCarthy 1977). To illustrate, he cites the case of a 13-year-old boy in New York who was charged with discharging a firearm with the intent to injure another (*In re Dimaggio* 1946). Even though it was clearly established that the child had no intent to shoot the victim—that the child was simply playing with his father's gun when the weapon discharged by accident—the court adjudicated the child delinquent, finding that the child had violated a law proscribing possession of a firearm without a license. Of course, this is an old decision, predating *Gault* by more than 20 years and may not reflect the manner in which *mens rea* issues would be dealt with today.

The Infancy Defense

As discussed above, the defense of infancy developed at common law to protect against the conviction and punishment of offenders who, by virtue of their immaturity, were presumed to be incapable of choosing to do wrong. Like the insanity defense, with which it shared a common purpose if not a common heritage (Fox 1970), the infancy defense fell into disuse with the rise of the juvenile court. In a sense, the idea of the juvenile court was conceived as an extension of the infancy defense, to ensure that persons below a certain age were shielded from criminal prosecution. Therefore, not only was the infancy defense seen as unnecessary—even redundant—in this new, paternalistic environment, but its use was regarded as subversive. "[A]ssertion of the defense could be viewed as wrongfully precluding treatment for those very children most susceptible to the benefits of intervention, children who had committed wrongs without a clear sense of the wrongfulness of their acts" (Walkover 1984, p. 516). Perhaps because, unlike the insanity defense (the successful use of which invariably results in treatment), the infancy defense does in fact preclude intervention, the defense has been slow to gain acceptance in the new, "criminalized" juvenile court. Indeed, nearly every court that has considered the matter in recent years has rejected the defense for use in juvenile court.

"Reliance on the rehabilitative ideal as the justifying spirit of a separate juvenile court threads its way through the reported cases denying use of the infancy defense" (Walkover 1984, p. 549). For example, in *In the Interest of Dow* (1979), an Illinois Court acknowledged that the consequences of a delinquency proceeding in juvenile court may not be "devoid of penal characteristics" but nevertheless found sufficient differences between criminal and juvenile proceedings to conclude that delinquency proceedings "are protective, not penal" and on this basis rejected application of the infancy defense for two preteens charged with aggravated battery. A Maryland court based its rejection of the infancy defense for a 13-year-old car thief on a finding that "by raising to eighteen the age below which a person is conclusively presumed to be incapable of committing a crime, the legislature implicitly repealed the infancy defense" (*In re Davis* 1973).

In New York, the infancy defense was deemed superfluous

in the case of a nine-year-old bank robber in light of the requirement that *mens rea* be established for adjudication of delinquency (*Matter of Robert M* 1981).

> [I]f the respondent offered evidence that any combination of factors, including immaturity, negates requisite specific intent, he will be exonerated unless his evidence is overcome beyond reasonable doubt. The application of these principles protects against imposition of undeserved punishment upon those who are "developmentally abnormal" or "grossly immature" without imposing a Common Law presumption which is inappropriate in the usual case and inconsistent with the legislative scheme for the adjudication of juvenile offense. (*Matter of Robert M* 1981, p. 863)

The infancy defense has been approved for use in juvenile court in very few reported cases. In one of these cases, *In re Gladys R* (1970), the California Supreme Court based its approval on a strict, technical construction of unique statutory language; thus, this decision should have little significance outside California (Walkover 1984, p. 553). In a second case, *Commonwealth v. Durham* (1978), the Pennsylvania Supreme Court ruled that for children between the ages of 7 and 14, criminal capacity, like *mens rea*, was an element of crime that had to be proved beyond a reasonable doubt in every case as a matter of constitutional due process. Nowhere else, however, has criminal capacity been viewed as an element of crime; thus, *Durham* is unlikely to have precedential value either (Walkover 1984, p. 554). Finally, in *In re Andrew M* (1977), the New York Family Court approved of the defense of infancy based on the simple reasoning that, because the purpose of the juvenile court in New York in fact no longer was exclusively protective, the rationale for denying the Common Law defense of infancy was lost.

> If we view juvenile proceedings as the Supreme Court does in *Gault* . . . and *Matter of Winship* . . . as being a special category of "almost criminal" liability, the fiction of a conclusive presumption of incapacity to commit a crime becomes a historical

vestige with roots in pre-*Gault* philosophy which falls in the face of the reality of minimum periods of secure incarceration newly enacted in the Juvenile Justice Reform Act of 1976. . . . With this reality in mind, the rebuttable presumption of incapacity, ostensibly swallowed within the conclusive presumption enacted by the Family Court Act, takes on new relevance. For, if the presumption which purports to absorb is illusory, how can it destroy by sheer inference the substantive defense of infancy available via the Command Law rebuttable presumption? (*In re Andrew M* 1977, p. 826)

At least one scholar, Andrew Walkover, has written passionately in support of allowing the infancy defense in juvenile court, arguing that, in fact, blame for culpable conduct is at the heart of every delinquency adjudication. "That both the *mens rea* requirement and the insanity defense continue to play a vital role in juvenile justice proceedings lends weight to the conclusion that the exercise of juvenile court jurisdiction over minor offenders must include consideration of the culpable conduct requirement" (Walkover 1984, p. 550). McCarthy provides support for this view, observing that "[i]f a child honestly thought that he was entering his grandmother's house, for instance, when in fact the child was entering the home of another, it would seem unlikely that any juvenile court would find him delinquent based on an unlawful entry" (McCarthy 1977, p. 194). Of course, the distinction between such innocent mistakes of fact and wrongful acts committed by children unable to distinguish good from evil is great. Although the offender who is operating under a simple mistake of fact and inadvertently commits a wrongful act presumably is unlikely to make the same mistake again and, thus, raises little call for alarm, the individual who was unable to distinguish right from wrong at the time that he or she violated the law is likely to be seen as a significant concern for public safety. Of course, if the child's inability to distinguish right from wrong has its basis in mental disorder, the public may be protected by finding the child legally insane and requiring the child to receive treatment for his or her disorder. If, on the other hand, the inability is due solely to the immaturity of the child, no mechanism is available to prevent the child from offending again. Because such a circumstance is difficult for our safety-conscious society to accept, particularly where the wrongful act is a violent one, it is unlikely that the defense of infancy ever will gain general acceptance in American juvenile courts, regardless of the cogency of legal arguments advanced in support of the doctrine.

Conclusion

The image of the juvenile court as a grand, benevolent child guidance clinic has lost all credibility in the last 20 years. Indeed, it is widely accepted today that retribution is one of the primary purposes of the juvenile court in America. In this climate, it is not surprising that questions of competency to stand trial and criminal responsibility show signs of vitality.

Given the emphasis that has been placed on procedural fairness in the juvenile court since the United States Supreme Court's decision in *In re Gault*, it would be difficult to deny the applicability of the doctrine of competency to stand trial in delinquency proceedings. If the child has the right to participate in these proceedings, as, of course, he or she does, then, for that right to have meaning, the child must be able to understand the proceedings and use them to his or her advantage.

In a similar vein, given the potentially punitive quality of delinquency dispositions in the juvenile court, one cannot with a clear conscience deny the delinquency defendant access to responsibility defenses that are available to adult criminal defendants. To suggest that the insanity defense is superfluous because the child who suffers from a mental disorder will receive treatment whether or not he or she is found insane ignores other potentially undesirable effects of a delinquency adjudication. Moreover, the child who is adjudicated delinquent despite his or her nonresponsibility has no guarantee of freedom should the symptoms of mental disorder remit.

Whether the infancy defense has a legitimate place in the juvenile court is debatable. Although the evidence is undeniable that delinquency dispositions frequently are punitive, this evidence is largely, if not exclusively, derived from cases in which the child was over the age of six. Accordingly, it may be true that for younger children, whom the infancy defense conclusively presumes to be incapable of crime, the juvenile justice system is not punitive and, thus, the infancy defense is unnecessary. For those over six, whom the infancy defense rebuttably presumes to be incapable, an arguably equivalent defense may be found in the concept of *mens rea*. If it is true that *mens rea* must be established by the state before a child may be adjudicated delinquent, then, to the extent that capacity is subsumed by *mens rea*, the defense of infancy is redundant. Of course, *mens rea* and capacity are not defined identically; thus, it is not clear that capacity in fact *is* subsumed by *mens rea*. Accordingly, there may be cases for which the infancy defense remains necessary, for example, the seven-year-old charged with murder who intended to kill but who, because of immaturity, did not appreciate the wrongfulness of the act.

In any event, whether the juvenile court will entertain questions of competency to stand trial, legal insanity, *mens rea*, or infancy may be a matter of relatively small proportion. Except in the most extraordinary of cases, it is unlikely that any of these issues has *great* outcome significance in the juvenile court. Accordingly, although the mental health professional who works with children should be aware of these issues and should be prepared to address them in court, he or she should not be distracted by these issues from the far more important question of disposition. Without a doubt, the most significant contribution that the mental health community can make to the juvenile justice process is to identify the needs of troubled youths and to provide services responsive to those needs. For these concerns to be lost in a battle over the niceties of legal doctrine would be tragic, indeed.

References

American Law Institute Model Penal Code Sec. 4.01 (official draft, 1962)

Breed v. Jones, 421 U.S. 519, 1975

Commonwealth v. Durham, 255 Pa. Super. 539, 1978

Dusky v. United States, 362 U.S. 402, 1960

Favole R: Mental disability in the American criminal process: four issue survey, in Mentally Disordered Offenders: Perspectives from Law and Social Science. Edited by Monahan J, Steadman H. New York, Plenum, 1983

Ford v. State, 1 Ga. 63, 25 S.E. 845, 1891

Fox SJ: Responsibility in the juvenile court. William and Mary Law Review 11:659–684, 1970

Grisso T, Miller MO, Sales B: Competency in juvenile court. International Journal of Law and Psychiatry 10:1–20, 1987

In re Andrew M, 398 N.Y.S. 2d 824, 1977

In re Causey, 363 So. 2d 472, La., 1978

In re C.W.M., 407 A.2d 617, D.C., 1979

In re Davis, 299 A.2d 856, 1973

In re Dimaggio, 65 N.Y.S. 2d 613, Dom. Rel. Ct. Kings County, 1946

In re Gault, 387 U.S. 1, 1967

In re Gladys R, 1 Cal. 3d 855, 1970

In re Glassberg, 230 La. 395, 88 So. 2d 707, 1956

In re H.C., 106 N.J. Super. 583, 256 A.2d 322, 1969

In re R.G.W., 342 A. 2d 869, 1975

In re Winship, 397 U.S. 358, 1970

In the Interest of Dow, 393 N.E. 2d 1346, 1979

Jackson v. Indiana, 406 U.S. 715, 1972

Jones v. United States, 103 S. Ct. 3043, 1983

Kolvin I: Studies in the childhood psychoses: diagnostic criteria and classification. Br J Psychiatry 118:381–389, 1971

Matter of Robert M, 441 N.Y.S. 2d 860, 1981

McCarthy FB: The role of the concept of responsibility in juvenile delinquency proceedings. Journal of Law Reform 10:181–219, 1977

President's Commission on Law Enforcement and Administration of Justice: Task Force Report: Juvenile Delinquency and Youth Crime. Washington, DC, U.S. Government Printing Office, 1967

Society for the Prevention of Pauperism in the City of New York: Report on the subject of erecting a house of refuge for vagrant and depraved young people, 1823. Reprinted in McCarthy FB: The role of the concept of responsibility in juvenile delinquency proceedings. Journal of Law Reform 10:188, 1977.

Stone A: The insanity defense on trial. Hosp Community Psychiatry 33:634–640, 1982

Walkover A: The infancy defense in the new juvenile court. UCLA Law Review 31:503–562, 1984

Warren JI, Fitch WL: Forensic evaluation in the community: an analysis of 475 referrals. Unpublished manuscript, 1987

Weissman JC: Toward an integrated theory of delinquency responsibility. Denver Law Journal 60:485–518, 1983

Winburn v. Wisconsin, 145 N.W. 2d 178, 184, 1966.d 178, 184, 1966

Chapter 7

Legal Outcome of Juveniles Charged with Homicide

DEWEY G. CORNELL, Ph.D.
LOIS STARESINA, A.M.L.S.
ELISSA P. BENEDEK, M.D.

Chapter 7

Legal Outcome of Juveniles Charged with Homicide

Extreme variation exists among the legal dispositions of juvenile homicide offenders. This variability is demonstrated by Cormier and Markus's (1980) review of 41 boys (ages 14 to 17 years) charged with murder or manslaughter in Montreal. Outcomes ranged from placement with relatives to life sentences. Most of the youths (61 percent) were retained in juvenile court, and these youths received rather benign treatment relative to the severity of their alleged offenses. Nearly half were not adjudicated delinquent, and the maximum available sentence for the remainder was confinement until age 21. Those youths who were transferred to adult court typically received much more severe dispositions; almost all were convicted and over half received life sentences.

The Philadelphia Study

Eigen's study (1981) of all 154 juveniles arrested for homicides in Philadelphia in 1970 offers some insight into the relationship between legal outcome and offender/offense characteristics. It should be noted that the 154 arrests involved only 63 homicides, and that most of the youths were charged as accessories rather than direct perpetrators of the homicides. However, Eigen's study raises a number of important and provocative points about the legal treatment of juvenile murderers; therefore, it will be reviewed in some detail.

165

Eigen reported that 75 of the youths were transferred to adult court, whereas 79 were retained under juvenile jurisdiction. As with the Montreal cases, the jurisdictional question was critical to eventual disposition. For a youth retained in juvenile court, "the maximum sentence is incarceration until the youth is 21; in criminal court, the maximum sentence is death" (p. 1082).

Several factors may predispose the court to transfer a youth to adult court. Eigen compared the relative incidence of four such "risk factors" in juveniles who were retained or transferred. He hypothesized that youths were at higher risk for transfer if they were: 1) 17 years old (approaching the age of majority); 2) had a previous criminal record; 3) personally inflicted the wound; and 4) were black *and* killed a white victim. Eigen found only equivocal evidence that these factors were predictive of transfer to adult court. For example, the few youths with three or more risk factors were somewhat more likely to be transferred than retained. Unfortunately, Eigen failed to employ rigorous and more precise procedures that would have tested the risk factor hypothesis more definitively, such as discriminant function analysis and comparison of his findings to overall base rates for court transfer.

Legal outcomes for juveniles retained in juvenile court were predictably mild. Of the 79 arrested and detained as juveniles, 61 were adjudicated delinquent, and only about half (30) were committed to juvenile institutions. Legal outcomes for those tried in adult court were much more severe. Nearly 90 percent of the juveniles tried in criminal court were sentenced to prison.

There was no indication that juveniles transferred to adult courts were treated more leniently than adults with homicide charges. On the contrary, juveniles charged with non-felony-related homicides seemed to receive slightly harsher sentences than adults with similar homicides.

Eigen made the quite plausible assertion that juveniles who committed felony-related homicides were prosecuted more vigorously by the district attorney's office than those who committed homicides in association with an argument or interpersonal conflict. Juveniles charged with felony-related homicides faced more serious consequences for their crimes. Almost all of the youths charged with felony-related homicides were convicted and sentenced to prison, but many of those charged with non-felony-related homicides went free or received relatively mild sentences.

Finally, Eigen found disturbing evidence suggestive of racial bias in sentencing. Black youths seemed to receive more severe sentences when the victims were white than when they were black. Among the 42 cases in which a black youth killed another black person, none received life imprisonment (although one youth did receive the death penalty). In contrast, 10 of 19 cases in which a black youth killed a white victim resulted in a sentence of life imprisonment. However, definitive evidence of racial bias requires that studies control for other factors that might explain race differences. For example, white victims might involve a higher proportion of felony-related murders or stranger murders, whereas more of the black victims might be family members or acquaintances of the black offender.

Nevertheless, concerns about bias against black offenders have been raised by many others. In their review of 17 previous studies, Liska and Tausig (1979) concluded that race affected legal dispositions for juvenile offenders even after controlling for prior record and seriousness of the offense. In more recent research, Bortner et al. (1985) found more equivocal results; after the juvenile system in one city stopped institutionalization of status offenders, there was a higher juvenile detention rate for blacks than for whites, but whites seemed to receive more severe dispositions. Juvenile court practices that reflect bias toward blacks may vary as a function of the severity of the offense. Because homicide is the most serious of crimes and has the most serious punitive consequences, research specific to the legal treatment of black juvenile homicide offenders is needed.

Other Outcome Research

Although conviction rates may be higher for youths transferred to adult court than for those retained in juvenile court, this may be an artifact of selecting the more serious and unequivocal cases for transfer. Findings in support of this hypothesis have been presented by Rudman et al. (1986) in a study of 138 youths charged with violent crimes in three urban areas. Rudman and colleagues compared transferred and retained youths after excluding youths who had not been *considered* for transfer to adult court. They found nearly identical conviction rates for the 67 youths transferred to adult court (92.2 percent) and the 71 who were retained in juvenile court (95.5 percent). These very high conviction rates are especially noteworthy in light of the authors' earlier report (Fagan et al. 1984). This report found an *overall* conviction rate of only 34.7 percent, irrespective of transfer consideration, for youths charged with the same types of offenses in the same court jurisdictions.

Rudman et al. (1986) predictably found that youths transferred to adult court were punished more severely than those retained in juvenile court. The discrepancy was most marked in homicide cases. Youths convicted in adult court received mean sentences of 247.5 months, as opposed to 55.7 months for the youths retained in juvenile courts. Similarly, Rosner and colleagues (1979) found a high conviction and imprisonment rate among adolescent murderers tried in New York adult courts.

Legal Outcomes for Michigan Youths

We attempted to determine the legal outcome for the 72 youths charged with homicide who were described in Chapter 3. Tracking down these cases proved much more difficult than we anticipated. They were referred from across the state of Michigan and the quality of court record-keeping varied widely from district to district. In addition, the study of juvenile homicide is such a politically sensitive subject that it was sometimes difficult to gain access to records. The subject is particularly sensitive in Detroit, where the overall homicide rate is high and juvenile homicide in particular is a frequent topic in the local news.

Follow-up information was obtained by a variety of methods, but primarily by contacting the court of disposition for each case. In some cases information was available more directly through the local prosecutor's office and, on occasion, from the defense counsel. Records were often difficult to locate. One case created a minor panic in the prosecutor's office when no disposition information could be found, and contact with prison authorities revealed no trace of the youth. Eventually, the youth was found to be incarcerated under a different name than appeared on the original court papers.

It bears repeating that this sample does not represent the broad population of all juveniles charged with homicide, but rather those referred for pretrial evaluation. The 72 adolescents who were evaluated at the Michigan Center for Forensic Psychiatry were referred primarily for two reasons: evaluation of competency to stand trial and/or criminal responsibility. Some of the youths were referred for evaluation of their fitness for waiver to adult court, but most had already been waived by the time of their referral to the Forensic Center. It may be that many juvenile courts in Michigan do not recognize that the Forensic Center can be a resource for juvenile waiver evaluations (in addition to competency and criminal responsibility evaluations) and may be more likely to rely on local resources.

Competency to Stand Trial

As discussed by Fitch in Chapter 6, competency to stand trial is a legal issue not commonly applied to juveniles, because the juvenile court usually takes a benign, protective stance toward youths and attempts to act in their best interests. Nevertheless, when youths commit serious crimes such as homicide, the process becomes more prosecutorial, and the need for the juvenile to defend himself or herself becomes more important. Of course, the emphasis on prosecution and defense is unequivocal if the youth is waived to adult court.

Michigan law, like many other states, defines competency to stand trial with wording very similar to that provided in the Dusky standard (Grisso 1986). Section 1020 (1) of the Michigan Mental Health Code states, in part:

> A defendant to a criminal charge shall be presumed competent to stand trial. He shall be determined incompetent to stand trial only if he is incapable because of his mental condition of understanding the nature and object of the proceedings against him or of assisting in his defense in a rational manner. The court shall determine the capacity of a defendant to assist in his defense by his ability to perform the tasks reasonably necessary for him to perform in the preparation of his defense and during the trial.

Fifty of the 72 referrals to the Forensic Center for pretrial evaluation included the question of competency to stand trial. All were referred after being waived to the adult court. Only three of the adolescents were recommended as incompetent to stand trial by the examining clinician, and all were adjudicated incompetent by the court. In no case did the court disagree with the clinician's recommendation. (Disagreements between the court and Forensic Center on matters of competency to stand trial in other cases are unusual, but not nonexistent.)

All three youths who were recommended as incompetent to stand trial were overtly psychotic at the time of their pretrial evaluation. A brief case description serves as an example:

> Sixteen-year-old Billy was charged with the murder of his best friend, whom he shot without warning one day at school. Upon clinical evaluation, Billy presented as paranoid and delusional. He reported that he was the subject of abuse and disrespect by his peers, and that he shot his friend out of jealousy because he was so popular. Billy complained that other kids teased him, but not his friend. He acknowledged planning the murder in great detail over a period of weeks. Billy made peculiar state-

ments in the courtroom and voiced paranoid delusions about the jury and his attorney, all of which supported the recommendation that he was incompetent to stand trial. Billy was given a diagnosis of schizophreniform disorder, hospitalized, and treated with medication and supportive individual therapy. Eventually, his delusions about his legal circumstances subsided and he showed sufficient improvement to be considered competent to stand trial.

Further information on this case is reported in the following section on criminal responsibility.

Criminal Responsibility

Michigan law. Criminal responsibility refers to the question of whether the defendant should be held blameworthy for an offense or exculpated as legally insane. Michigan law (Chapter 8, Section 21a, Act 180 of the Public Acts of 1975) follows the recommendations of the American Law Institute in defining insanity, which have been adopted by many other states:

> (1) A person is legally insane if, as a result of mental illness as defined in Section 400a . . . , or as a result of mental retardation as defined in Section 500 . . . , that person lacks substantial capacity either to appreciate the wrongfulness of his conduct or to conform his conduct to the requirements of the law.
> (2) A person who is under the influence of voluntarily consumed or injected alcohol or controlled substances at the time of his alleged offense shall not thereby be deemed to have been legally insane.

Mental illness is defined as "a substantial disorder of thought or mood which significantly impairs judgment, behavior, capacity to recognize reality, or ability to cope with the ordinary demands of life" (Section 400a of Act 158 of the Michigan Public Acts of 1974). This definition is most commonly interpreted to mean psychosis, although other conditions (for example, severe depression) may be included.

By Michigan law, which is similar to laws in most other

states, defendants who are acquitted as not guilty by reason of insanity are not hospitalized for involuntary psychiatric *treatment*; instead, they are committed (usually to the Forensic Center) for 60 days of diagnostic *evaluation*. At the conclusion of this time they are reviewed by the probate court for involuntary civil commitment, which in essence requires the presence of a mental disorder with indications of imminent dangerousness to self or others. If acquittees do not meet civil commitment criteria, there is no legal alternative to releasing them.

Michigan insanity cases. Sixty-three youths were evaluated for criminal responsibility. In the opinion of the forensic examiners, only one youth met the criteria for legal insanity. Three youths were adjudicated not guilty by reason of insanity, including the one identified by the forensic examiner. Therefore, overall agreement between forensic examiners and the courts was 96.8 percent (61 of 63 cases).

The youth who was recommended as meeting the insanity criteria (previously described in Chapter 2) was clearly extremely disturbed:

At age 17 Allen had already been hospitalized several times for psychotic episodes that included auditory hallucinations, delusions, and formal thought disorder. In addition, he had a history of aggressive behavior that included attempting to drown his siblings. He stabbed a friend to death with a hunting knife, and later reported that he had heard the voice of God commanding him to kill his friend in order to free his friend's soul from his body and thereby save the world.

At the time of his forensic evaluation, Allen presented as grossly psychotic, claiming to be God and expressing himself in loose, fragmented statements with inappropriate affect. He was hospitalized as incompetent to stand trial and eventually restored to competency. He was adjudicated not guilty by reason of insanity and returned to the Forensic Center for the statutory 60-day evaluation period, followed by a civil court hearing that determined that he met criteria for involuntary commitment. Allen has continued to manifest psychotic symptoms, as well as dangerous behavior, and has been hospitalized now for more than 4 years.

The case of Allen contrasts sharply with those of the other two youths who were found not guilty by reason of insanity, contrary to the opinion of the Forensic Center examiners.

Seventeen-year-old Sonny was charged with the murder of a peer during a night when the two of them had been out drinking and smoking hashish with friends. The two of them had returned to his friend's house, where Sonny stabbed the victim over two dozen times. Coincidentally, Sonny was spotted by police leaving the house and questioned because he was splattered with blood. He initially reported that he had been in a bar fight, but when police grew suspicious and found the body, he claimed that he had acted in self-defense.

One set of experts found that Sonny presented no symptoms of mental illness and assigned diagnoses of antisocial personality disorder and substance abuse. An opposing group diagnosed Sonny as having had a dissociative reaction, which one expert witness described as triggered by "subconscious homosexual feelings" associated with his troubled relationship with his father.

The jury acquitted Sonny as not guilty by reason of insanity and he was committed for 60 days of diagnostic evaluation. He spent most of the time reading and kept to himself. At the conclusion of the evaluation period, two independent examiners found no indication of current mental illness. At the civil court hearing, he was found not committable and released.

The third case of an insanity acquittal presents somewhat different reasons for a disagreement between the court and expert opinion:

Seventeen-year-old Fred shot and killed his father during one of a series of episodes in which his father physically abused his sister. Fred's father had an extensive history of abusing Fred, his siblings, and his mother.

The forensic examiner testified in court about Fred's traumatic experiences and the effect his father had on him, but did not feel that Fred could be diagnosed as suffering from a "mental illness." Although technically Fred did not appear to meet the legal criteria for insanity, he was exculpated by the jury and remanded to the Forensic Center for diagnostic observation. At the conclusion of the evaluation period, the civil court found no grounds for civil commitment and he was released.

Undoubtedly the jury's sympathetic reaction to Fred played some role in its decision making. From a juror's lay perspective, Fred's reaction to his father during yet another episode of witnessing physical abuse might well invoke intuitive notions of "temporary insanity." However, this conception of insanity as a "heat-of-passion" reaction to severe stress is qualitatively different from the kind of case represented by Allen. Fred did not suffer from schizophrenia or any similar mental disorder; he did not even profess amnesia for the offense or give any indication that he acted in a dissociated state. Moreover, Fred did not deny the intentional nature of his behavior or his awareness that his actions were wrong. However justifiable the offense might appear from some larger moral perspective, it is far from clear that the insanity statute represented the appropriate legal resolution.

Guilty but mentally ill. In response to widespread public concern about the release of presumably dangerous insanity acquittees, Michigan devised a new option: the verdict of guilty but mentally ill (GBMI) (Michigan Acts 179 and 180 of the Public Acts of 1975; 70 Michigan Compiled Laws Annotated 786,36(1)). In essence, this verdict applies to defendants who meet the criterion of mental illness (or mental retardation, which is termed GBMR) under the insanity statute, but fail to meet either the cognitive or the volitional prong of the second criterion (lacking substantial capacity either to appreciate wrongfulness or to conform conduct). Various forms of a GBMI verdict have been adopted in approximately a dozen other states (Blunt and Stock 1985).

The GBMI verdict has in many ways not lived up to

expectations and has been quite controversial (Blunt and Stock 1985). Although the GBMI verdict may be appealing in that it appears to strike a compromise between the full responsibility assigned to the convicted and absence of responsibility awarded to the acquitted, in practical terms the GBMI verdict is a form of outright conviction. The defendent found GBMI is convicted of the offense and can be sentenced in exactly the same way as an ordinary conviction. The GBMI verdict simply acknowledges the presence of mental illness and indicates the potential need for mental health treatment. Of course, anyone convicted of a crime and sentenced to prison has a right to treatment of his or her mental illness, whether or not it was evident at the time of the offense.

Three defendants evaluated for criminal responsibility and recommended as responsible (not insane) were convicted as GBMI. One of the cases was described in the section on competency:

> Sixteen-year-old Billy, who had shot his friend and later showed paranoid symptoms, had been found incompetent to stand trial and clearly was mentally ill. This mental illness was present at the time of the offense, so that he met the first criterion for insanity. However, his prolonged planning of the offense, deliberate behavior, and acknowledged awareness of its wrongfulness apparently ruled out an insanity acquittal. Nevertheless, the jury found him GBMI for second degree murder and he was sentenced to 20 years in prison. Subsequently, his condition worsened and he was hospitalized while in prison with a diagnosis of schizophrenia.

The remaining two youths had committed homicides while intoxicated on drugs. They were excluded from the insanity defense because Michigan law (quoted above) does not permit exculpation based on voluntary intoxication. One youth was grossly psychotic on PCP and stabbed his brother to death in response to a hallucinated command from God and the delusional belief that he was killing the Antichrist. He was found GBMI of second degree murder and sentenced to 4 to 15 years in prison.

The other case was more equivocal. The youth gained entry to a house by asking for a drink of water and then assaulted the babysitter. He was observed by a child and fled the scene. Later, he claimed amnesia for the offense. The Forensic Center clinician diagnosed him as having an antisocial personality disorder and substance abuse problems. Another examiner concluded that the youth's lack of memory indicated that he was psychotic and recommended that he met criteria for insanity. The youth agreed to a plea bargain of GBMI to second degree murder and was sentenced to 10 to 20 years.

Adolescents Retained in Juvenile Court

In Michigan, the age of legal majority for criminal prosecution is 17; that is, adolescents are charged and prosecuted as adults when they reach the age of 17. Adolescents 15 and 16 years old can be waived to adult court, based on a hearing conducted in the juvenile court and decided by the juvenile court judge. The criteria for waiver have been modified slightly over the years of this study, but generally include the following broad factors:

1. the juvenile's prior record, character, and maturity;
2. the seriousness of the offense;
3. the juvenile's amenability to rehabilitation;
4. the suitability of available programs and facilities; and
5. the interests of public welfare and safety (Michigan Juvenile Court Rules 1987).

Adolescents 14 years and younger cannot be waived to adult court and therefore must remain under juvenile court jurisdiction.

Because of Michigan's relatively low age for adult status, the majority of adolescents in this sample (49 of 72, 68 percent) were charged at the outset in adult court. Twenty youths (28 percent) were eligible for waiver. Data on 19 of these youths were available, and almost all of these were waived to adult court jurisdiction (18 of 19, 95 percent).

176

The single 15-year-old youth who was considered for waiver, but not waived, was involved in a controversial case evaluated by a series of forensic examiners:

Johnny shot and killed his father after an argument in which his father called him names and made fun of him. A few moments later he shot and killed his mother as well.

Johnny had an extensive history of adjustment problems and involvement with juvenile authorities before the homicide. He made failing grades in school and was frequently in trouble for behavior problems that included fighting with peers and vandalism. He was reported to use marijuana and other drugs. Johnny had frequent arguments with both his mother and father and had been known to threaten them. His father was described as a strict disciplinarian and perfectionist who frequently derided his son as incompetent or inadequate and also physically abused him on many occasions. The father was reported to have sexually abused several of his children, including Johnny, several years prior to the offense.

Johnny was evaluated by a series of forensic examiners who arrived at different conclusions. Some regarded him as suffering from a severe character disorder, experiencing no remorse for his actions, and suitable for waiver to adult court. Others found Johnny to have serious personality problems, but to be remorseful for the offense and amenable to treatment by psychotherapy. All agreed that Johnny was not psychotic presently, but one examiner saw his explosive reaction to his father as a form of "temporary insanity." A complete neurological evaluation that included a CT scan and EEG was negative.

Johnny was not waived to adult court. He was adjudicated in juvenile court and placed in a boys' training school, to be released at age 19.

There were three youths ages 12 to 14 who could not be considered for waiver. The youngest was a 12-year-old who stabbed a peer multiple times but insisted that it was an accident. Another was a 14-year-old who brutally attacked and killed an elderly female neighbor with a club. His motive was never clear, although she had been disrobed and he may have intended a sexual assault. The third boy was 13 years old when he killed an elderly woman who had the misfortune to return home while he was committing a burglary. When discovered, he attempted to subdue her by striking her on the head with a heavy object.

Adolescents Tried in Adult Court

A total of 67 adolescents (ages 15–18 at the time of offense) charged with homicide were tried in the adult criminal courts. As indicated in Table 1, almost three-quarters of them were

TABLE 1. Adolescents tried for murder in Michigan adult courts: age and group comparisons

Variable	All cases (%)	Age comparison		Group comparison	
		15–16	17–18	Crime	Conflict
Initial charge					
First degree	49 (73)	13	36	33	13
Second degree	7 (10)	1	6	0	5
Open (unspecified)	11 (16)	4	7	3	8
Type of trial					
Bench trial	43 (68)	9	34	24	15
Jury trial	20 (32)	8	12	9	10
Plea bargain					
Yes	25 (42)	5	20	13	10
No	35 (58)	11	24	19	13
Outcome					
Acquitted or dismissed	8 (13)	0	8	2	5
Convicted	55 (87)	17	38	31	20
Conviction charge					
First degree	21 (38)	8	13	14	7
Second degree	29 (53)	8	21	16	10
Manslaughter	5 (9)	1	4	1	3
Sentence					
Not convicted	8 (13)	0	8	2	5
Probation	1 (2)	1	0	0	1
Less than 10 years	9 (14)	2	7	3	4
10 or more years	26 (41)	7	19	15	9
Natural life	19 (30)	7	12	13	6

Note. $n = 67$ for initial charges, but some cases missing or pending outcome data for remaining variables. Maximum $n = 62$ for crime and conflict groups because five psychotic group cases are omitted.

charged with first degree murder. Almost two-thirds of the youths elected a bench trial rather than a trial by jury. This proportion is so large probably because it included 25 youths who pled guilty in a plea bargain arrangement. The penalty for conviction on first degree murder in Michigan is natural life (that is, life imprisonment without parole), which undoubtedly provided considerable incentive for defendants to plead guilty to second degree murder. Almost all of the youths were convicted; only 8 cases (13 percent) resulted in dismissal or acquittal.

Prison sentences for convicted adolescents varied from 1 youth who received probation to 19 who received the maximum life sentence. Overall, nearly three-quarters of the convicted youths received a sentence of 10 or more years. (We attempted to determine more precisely how much time an individual would serve for sentences designating a specific term of years. However, a more detailed determination proved impossible. Michigan prison sentences and parole policies are governed by a complex series of rules that have many exceptions, and these rules are applied on a case-by-case basis.)

Michigan-Philadelphia comparisons. Some comparisons between Michigan data (Table 1) and Philadelphia data can be made, although differences in sample selection and coding procedures, as well as differences in state laws, complicate the picture. The 87 percent Michigan conviction rate is remarkably similar to the 89 percent rate in Philadelphia (Eigen 1981). However, most Philadelphia youths appear to have been treated more leniently by the courts, with 12 percent receiving probation or no sentence, and only 14 percent receiving a sentence of more than 12 years. In contrast, the majority of Michigan youth (45 of 55, 82 percent) received a sentence of 10 or more years.

Several factors complicate the Michigan-Philadelphia comparison and make straightforward conclusions difficult. First, the Philadelphia study included youths charged as accessories to murder, whereas in the Michigan study virtually all of

179

the youths were alleged to have participated directly in the murder. (Almost all confessed explicitly to carrying out the murder during their Forensic Center evaluation.) Second, sentencing alternatives differ dramatically between Michigan and Philadelphia. The state of Pennsylvania permits capital punishment, whereas Michigan was the first state to move to abolish the death penalty, with its first action taken in 1847 and complete abolition in 1963 (Michigan Public Act 119 of 1963). Moreover, Michigan mandates a natural life sentence for conviction on first degree murder, whereas Pennsylvania does not. Finally, sentences designated as a term of years are difficult to interpret because differing parole policies determine how much of a sentence will be served.

Age comparisons.   The younger adolescents (ages 15–16) who were transferred into adult court were compared to those defendants (ages 17–18) initially charged as adults. There was no evidence that adolescents transferred into the adult court were treated any more leniently than the older youths who originally were charged as adults. As shown in Table 2, the majority of both groups were charged with first degree murder and elected a bench trial. Although proportionately more older than younger youths elected a bench trial, the difference was not significant ($p = 0.10$ by Fisher exact test). The few youths who were not convicted all came from the larger group of older defendants, but this contrast fell short of significance ($p = 0.07$ by Fisher exact test).

There were no large discrepancies between groups in whether the youths were convicted of first degree murder, second degree murder, or manslaughter, although the limited distribution of cases precluded significance testing. If anything, there may have been a tendency for the younger youths to receive *harsher* sentences than their older counterparts, because a larger proportion (7 of 17, 41 percent) of the younger adolescents received life sentences than did the older group (10 of 38, 26 percent). To test this hypothesis further, we rank ordered outcomes from least to most severe: acquittal or dismissal of charges, conviction with probation, prison sentence less than 10 years, prison sentence of 10 or more years, and life sentence. However, a rank-order, nonparametric test of sentencing differences between age groups also fell short of significance (Mann-Whitney $U = 299$, $p = 0.13$).

Crime and conflict group comparisons. Finally, we returned to our previous distinction between crime and conflict youth (see Chapter 3). As described in Table 2, the majority of youth in both groups declined to plea bargain, but opted for a bench trial rather than a jury trial. There were no significant differences between groups in these decisions. Most of the youth in both groups were charged with first degree murder, and almost all of those in both groups were convicted. Slightly more defendants in the crime group (31 of 33, 94 percent) were convicted than in the conflict group (20 of 25, 80 percent), but the difference was not significant ($p = 0.11$ by Fisher exact test).

There was some indication that youths in the crime group were treated more severely than those in the conflict group. When outcomes were again rank ordered from least severe to most severe, there was a significant tendency for crime group youths to be treated more harshly (Mann-Whitney $U = 292$, $p = 0.046$).

Conclusion

Juveniles charged with homicide face a wide variety of legal outcomes. The single most important determining factor appears to be the decision to transfer the juvenile to adult court, because of the adult court's far greater latitude in dispositions, the full range of which clearly is used in sentencing youths charged with homicide. An important direction for future research would be to examine the factors associated with transfer decisions for juvenile homicide cases. Once juveniles are transferred to adult court, there is no evidence that they are treated more leniently than slightly older defendants (although comparisons with much older defendants remain unexamined).

The classification of defendants into crime and conflict groups bears a modest relationship to legal outcome; more specific factors concerning the circumstances of the offense are nested within this distinction and remain to be examined in more detail.

References

Blunt LW, Stock HV: Guilty but mentally ill: an alternative verdict. Behavioral Sciences and the Law 3:49–67, 1985

Bortner MA, Sunderland ML, Winn R: Race and the impact of juvenile deinstitutionalization. Crime and Delinquency 31(1):35–46, 1985

Cormier B, Markus B: A longitudinal study of adolescent murderers. Bull Am Acad Psychiatry Law 8:240–260, 1980

Eigen JP: Punishing youth homicide offenders in Philadelphia. Journal of Criminal Law and Criminology 72(3):1072–1093, 1981

Fagan J, Rudman C, Hartstone E: System processing of violent juvenile offenders: an empirical assessment, in Violent Juvenile Offenders: An Anthology. Edited by Mathias R, Demuro P, Allinson R, et al. Newark, NJ, National Council on Crime and Delinquency, 1984

Grisso T: Evaluating Competencies: Forensic Assessments and Instruments. New York, Plenum Press, 1986

Liska AE, Tausig M: Theoretical interpretations of sociological class and racial differentials in legal decision-making for juveniles. Sociological Quarterly 23(2):197–207, 1979

Michigan Juvenile Court Rules. Wilmette, IL, Callaghan & Company, 1987

Rosner R, Weiderlight M, Rosner M, et al: Adolescents accused of murder and manslaughter: a five year descriptive study. Bull Am Acad Psychiatry Law 7:342–351, 1970

Rudman C, Hartstone E, Fagan J, et al: Violent youth in adult court: process and punishment. Crime and Delinquency 32:75–96, 1986

Chapter 8

Juvenile Homicide: A Study in Legal Ambivalence

RICHARD J. BONNIE, L.L.B.

Chapter 8

Juvenile Homicide: A Study in Legal Ambivalence

Anglo-American penal law reflects an uneasy tension between two paradigmatic conceptions of the goals of the sentencing process. On the one side is what I will call the classical view. This approach emphasizes the nature and seriousness of the offense as the predominant consideration in criminal sentencing; under this view, an explicit connection between the severity of punishment and the seriousness of the offense is necessary to achieve the retributive and deterrent goals of the penal law. In its most pronounced form, this view is reflected in the imposition of mandatory sentences on all persons convicted of a particular type of offense.

On the other side is the philosophy of individualized sentencing; under this view, the social goal of preventing crime is thought to be served best by choosing the sentence most likely to minimize further criminality, either by facilitating rehabilitation or by incapacitating the offender. Whereas the classical view tends toward determinacy through the application of rules, an individualized system relies on discretionary decisions by sentencing judges and parole boards.

The twentieth-century history of sentencing reform reflects wide swings from one paradigm to the other. In 1949, for example, the U.S. Supreme Court, speaking through Justice Black (*Williams v. New York* 1949, pp. 248–249) took note of the ascendancy of the individualization paradigm:

The belief no longer prevails that every offense in a like legal category calls for an identical punishment without regard to the past life and habits of a particular offender. . . . Today's philosophy of individualizing sentences makes sharp distinctions for example between first and repeated offenders. Indeterminate sentences, the ultimate termination of which are sometimes decided by non-judicial agencies, have to a large extent taken the place of the old rigidly fixed punishments. . . . Retribution is no longer the dominant objective of the criminal law. Reformation and rehabilitation of offenders have become important goals of criminal jurisprudence.

At the time it was written, Justice Black's statement no doubt reflected the prevailing opinion not only of the judiciary, but also of experts in the fields of criminology and criminal law, and probably of the public at large. It no longer does. Instead, contemporary sentencing legislation reflects a marked shift toward the classical paradigm, now commonly characterized as a philosophy of "just desserts."

The ascendant opinion is emphatically reflected in the preamble to the California sentencing statute, enacted in 1976 (Cal. Penal Code, 1985): "The legislature finds and declares that the purpose of imprisonment for crime is punishment. This purpose is best served by terms proportionate to the seriousness of the offense with provision for uniformity in the sentences of offenders committing the same offense under similar circumstances." There is no room in this scheme for individualized, and ultimately discretionary, judgments regarding the offender's future behavior or the likely behavioral effects of alternative interventions.

Linking crime and punishment is not a mechanical task, of course, and many "dessert"-based sentencing schemes leave some room for discretionary judgments about offense seriousness and culpability and for variations based on the offender's prior record. Legislative judgments about the ranking of crimes and the level of punishment severity also differ. On one point, however, the contemporary generation of sentencing statutes reflects a uniform and long-standing judgment: intentional homicide is at the top of the scale of offense seriousness. Current statutes typically prescribe minimum sentences of imprisonment for the highest grade of murder, and mandatory terms of life imprisonment are not uncommon. Renewed emphasis on the retributive and deterrent goals of criminal punishment is reflected in the fact that 37 states now prescribe the death penalty for aggravated forms of intentional murder.

This marked shift in prevailing attitudes toward criminal punishment would appear to tug against the operating assumptions of the juvenile justice system. It has been said that the juvenile court, first established in the early decades of this century, "represents the most important and ambitious effort yet undertaken to give practical expression to the rehabilitative ideal"—the benevolent form of what I have characterized as the individualization paradigm (Allen 1964, pp. 48–49). To the founders of the juvenile court, the judge's goal was not to proclaim guilt but to ascertain "how [the offender] has become what he is, and what had best be done in his interest and in the interest of the state to save him from a downward career" (Mack 1909, pp. 119–120). Treatment, not punishment, is said to be the purpose of delinquency intervention, even today (*In re Davis* 1973).

It would be a mistake to assume, however, that the law has ever reflected an unequivocal commitment to the rehabilitative ideal as the preferred response to adolescent criminality. The jurisdiction of juvenile courts over adolescents charged with homicide and other serious offenses has been a subject of continuing controversy since these courts were first established (McKenna and Grossman 1942; O'Connel 1937). Indeed, most of the early statutes either excluded murder and other serious offenses from juvenile court jurisdiction, regardless of the offender's age, or permitted the prosecutor to evade the juvenile court by invoking the criminal court's jurisdiction directly in these cases (Barrows 1973).

As juvenile court legislation evolved during the middle of this century, the tension between the two paradigms was resolved by most legislatures in the following manner:

187

1. *Juvenile* court jurisdiction was exclusive, regardless of the offense, if the offender was younger than a designated age when the offense was committed, usually 14.
2. *Criminal* court jurisdiction was exclusive, regardless of offense, if the offender was older than a designated age when the offense was committed, typically 18.
3. If there was probable cause to believe that an offender between these jurisdictional ages had committed a felony, the juvenile court could "waive" its jurisdiction and transfer the case to the criminal court. This decision was to be based on an individualized judgment regarding whether the offender was "amenable" to treatment in the juvenile court.

These transfer mechanisms "permit a state to retain a higher maximum age of juvenile court jurisdiction while simultaneously allowing removal to adult criminal courts of those youths whose highly visible, serious, or repetitive criminality threatens community safety or stimulates public outrage" (Feld 1983, p. 196).

One cannot dip into the literature on adolescent crime or the juvenile justice system today without being struck by its concentration on "the violent juvenile." Ever since Wolfgang and his colleagues (1972) found, in their Philadelphia cohort study, that 6 percent of the cohort accounted for 52 percent of the crime committed by the cohort (including 55 percent of the violent offenses and all of the homicides), criminologists have been preoccupied with the effort to identify those factors that differentiate the "violent few" from their peers.

This pervasive concern about juvenile violence has turned up the heat on the simmering controversy regarding the mission and performance of the juvenile justice system. Doubts about the capacity of the juvenile system to protect the public from the "violent juvenile" have led to widespread efforts to shift jurisdiction of these cases entirely to the criminal courts. More sweeping reforms also have been proposed—proposals that call into question the basic premises, and continued existence, of the juvenile system itself.

The present controversy has its roots in the 1960s, when pervasive skepticism about the benevolent consequences of delinquency intervention led the Supreme Court to bring the procedures of the juvenile court into line with those governing the criminal process. As Justice Fortas put it (*Kent v. United States* 1966, p. 546), the offender processed in the juvenile court "receives the worst of both worlds: [he] gets neither the protections accorded to adults nor the solicitous care and regenerative treatment postulated for children." Moreover, the President's Commission on Law Enforcement and Administration of Justice observed in 1967:

> While statutes, judges and commentators still talk in the language of compassion, help and treatment, it has become clear that in fact the same purposes that characterize the use of the criminal law for adult offenders—retribution, condemnation, incapacitation—are involved in the disposition of juvenile offenders too. (p. 7)

The Supreme Court and the President's Commission emphasized the inevitable influence of retributive and deterrent considerations on the actual practices of the juvenile court. But neither of them questioned its basic premise; they sought to discipline the system, not to abolish it or abandon its decided tilt toward individualization. As the President's Commission put it, "what should distinguish the juvenile from the criminal courts is greater emphasis on rehabilitation, not exclusive preoccupation with it" (p. 9).

A decade later, however, the critics were not so restrained. As an influential task force established by the Twentieth Century Fund (1978) noted:

> The theory behind the juvenile court is not merely obsolete; it is a fairy tale that never came true. The court has helped some young offenders, but it has punished others. From the beginning, juvenile court judges have considered the interests of the state as well as those of the offender. It is pointless to pretend that social policy toward youth crime is based solely on the best

interests of the young offender or that the best interests of the offender and those of the state are always the same. (p. 6)

The task force recommended that the dispositional structure of the juvenile court be reformulated to echo the retributive premises of the criminal court, acknowledging that the justifying purpose of intervention is to punish the adolescent offender for intentionally wrongful behavior. Specifically, the task force declared that "the degree of punishment available for youth crime should be proportional to the seriousness of the offense" (p. 8). Two years later, the same view was reflected in the Juvenile Justice Standards promulgated by the Institute of Judicial Administration and the American Bar Association. Both reports set forth a scheme of presumptive sentences for juvenile offenses, although the range of prescribed sentences was markedly less severe than the range of penalties traditionally authorized for offenders convicted in criminal courts.

Such a fundamental reorientation of the juvenile justice system has been effected by legislation in only a few states. (See, for example, Minnesota, Washington.) However, heightened ambivalence about the underlying purposes of delinquency adjudication is strongly evident in active legislative reconsideration of the boundary between juvenile and criminal court jurisdiction in cases involving older adolescents charged with violent offenses.

As things now stand, the juvenile justice system, still tilted toward the individualization paradigm, operates side by side with a regime of criminal sentencing increasingly tilted toward the classical paradigm. Naturally, the tension between the two systems is greatest at the border between them and is especially pronounced (as has historically been the case) when the offender is charged with intentional homicide or other offenses involving serious violence. In the remainder of this chapter, I want to focus on what is perhaps the most significant decision made by the judicial system in a case involving a juvenile charged with homicide—whether he or she will be tried in juvenile or criminal court.

Table 1. Age at which offenders are subject to exclusive jurisdiction of the criminal court

Age (years)			
16	17	18	19
Connecticut	Georgia	Alabama	Wyoming
New York [a]	Hawaii	Alaska	
North Carolina [a]	Idaho	Arizona	
Vermont [b]	Illinois	Arkansas	
	Louisiana [c]	California	
	Massachusetts	Colorado	
	Michigan	Delaware [d]	
	Missouri	District of Columbia	
	South Carolina	Florida	
	Texas	Indiana [e]	
		Iowa	
		Kansas	
		Kentucky	
		Maine	
		Maryland [a]	
		Minnesota	
		Mississippi [f]	
		Montana	
		Nebraska	
		Nevada [d]	
		New Hampshire	
		New Jersey	
		New Mexico	
		North Dakota	
		Ohio	
		Oklahoma [e]	
		Oregon	
		Pennsylvania [b,d]	
		Rhode Island	
		South Dakota	
		Tennessee	
		Utah	
		Virginia	
		Washington	
		West Virginia	
		Wisconsin	
Total: 4	Total: 10	Total: 36	Total: 1

[a] 14 for murder and other serious offenses.
[b] Criminal court has authority to transfer the case to juvenile court.
[c] 15 for murder and other serious offenses.
[d] Criminal court has exclusive jurisdiction over murder cases.
[e] 16 for murder and other serious offenses.
[f] 13 for capital offenses.

Jurisdictional Structure Governing Adjudication of Youths Charged with Homicide

The circumstances under which a person under the age of 18 can be tried in criminal court vary widely from state to state. As Table 1 shows, the maximum age of juvenile court jurisdiction is less than 18 years in 14 states. Moreover, in 6 of the 37 states prescribing 18 (or 19) years as the generally applicable jurisdictional age, criminal court jurisdiction is mandatory for some younger offenders if they are charged with homicide or other serious offenses; these states have, in effect, selectively lowered the maximum age of juvenile court jurisdiction for those offenses.

Within the boundaries set by the maximum jurisdictional age of juvenile courts, most states *permit* criminal court jurisdiction in some category of cases involving youths below the maximum age. In some states, the choice of court is up to the prosecutor or the criminal court; however, in most states, the decision rests with the juvenile court judge (Snyder and Hutzler 1981). The ages at which youths charged with felonies (or some equivalent statutory category of offenses) become eligible for transfer to criminal court are depicted in Table 2. Note that transfer to criminal court is possible in most states if the offender was at least 14 at the time of the offense.

Even this does not complete the story, however. The age at which a case otherwise within the juvenile court jurisdiction may be transferred to criminal court is lowered even more in some jurisdictions for youths charged with murder (Table 3).

In summary, criminal court jurisdiction is *permitted* for juveniles charged with murder if they are 16 or 17 years old in every state and if they are 14 or 15 years old in most states. Although criminal court jurisdiction is either mandatory or within the discretion of the prosecutor or criminal court in some states (from one-fifth to two-fifths, depending on the offender's age), in most jurisdictions the jurisdictional decision lies entirely within the discretion of the juvenile court.

The juvenile court's discretion is relatively unconstrained

Table 2. Generally applicable minimum age for exercise of criminal court jurisdiction in felony cases (age at which waiver of juvenile court jurisdiction is possible)

		Age (years)			
None	10	13	14	15	16
Alaska	Vermont	Illinois	Alabama	Arkansas[a]	California
Arizona	South Dakota	Mississippi	Colorado	District of Columbia	Delaware
Maine			Connecticut[b]	Georgia	Hawaii
Nebraska[a]			Florida	Idaho	Indiana
New Hampshire			Iowa	Louisiana	Montana
Oklahoma			Kansas	Maryland	Nevada
Washington			Kentucky	Michigan	New Mexico
Wyoming[a]			Massachusetts	Ohio	North Dakota
			Minnesota	Texas	Oregon
			Missouri	Virginia	Rhode Island
			New Jersey		South Carolina
			New York[b]		Tennessee
			North Carolina		West Virginia
			Pennsylvania		Wisconsin
			Utah		
Total: 8	Total: 2	Total: 2	Total: 15	Total: 10	Total: 14

[a] Wholly in discretion of prosecutor.
[b] Criminal court jurisdiction is mandatory at this age.

193

Table 3. Minimum age for exercise of criminal court jurisdiction in murder cases

None	10	13	Age (years) 14	15	16
Alaska	Indiana [a]	Georgia [b]	Alabama	Arkansas	California
Arizona	South Dakota	Illinois	Colorado	District of Columbia	Delaware
Florida [c]	Vermont	Mississippi [d]	Connecticut	Idaho	Hawaii
Kentucky			Iowa	Louisiana [d]	Montana
Maine			Kansas	Michigan	North Dakota
Maryland [d]			Massachusetts	New Mexico	Oregon
Nebraska [c]			Minnesota	Ohio	Rhode Island
Nevada [d]			Missouri	Tennessee	Wisconsin
New Hampshire			New Jersey	Texas	
Oklahoma [a]			New York [d]	Virginia	
Pennsylvania [e]			North Carolina [d]		
South Carolina			Utah		
Washington					
West Virginia					
Wyoming [c]					
Total: 15	Total: 3	Total: 3	Total: 12	Total: 10	Total: 8

[a] Jurisdiction is exclusive if youth is 16.
[b] Judicial waiver is permitted if youth is 13, but prosecutor appears to have authority to invoke criminal court jurisdiction in any case.
[c] Prosecution has discretion to invoke criminal court jurisdiction.
[d] Criminal court jurisdiction is mandatory.
[e] Criminal court jurisdiction is mandatory, but criminal court may transfer case to juvenile court.

in most jurisdictions. The judge is typically directed to waive jurisdiction only upon finding that the juvenile is not amenable to treatment within the juvenile system. Because this inquiry is so highly discretionary, decisions to retain or waive jurisdiction are rarely reversed on appeal. However, in a few states (for example, California, Minnesota), the juvenile judge's discretion has been constrained recently by statutory presumptions linked to the offense charged and the offender's prior record.

The Significance of Jurisdictional Choice

On the face of the law, severe dispositional consequences turn on whether the adolescent charged with a violent offense is tried in juvenile or criminal court. Juvenile court records are insulated from the stigmatizing and often disabling uses to which records of criminal conviction can be put. (Critics of the juvenile court point out that transfer to criminal court may have an *advantage:* because of jury trial and heightened concern with procedural fairness, criminal court adjudication may reduce the risk of erroneous conviction.) More importantly, the maximum period of confinement to which the offender can be sentenced differs significantly: in the juvenile court, the court's jurisdiction (and hence the state's authority to intervene) expires when the offender reaches a designated age, typically 21; thus for older adolescents nearing the maximum age of juvenile court's adjudicatory jurisdiction (typically 18 years), the ceiling on confinement may be quite low (three or four years at most) as compared with the lengthy terms available to the criminal court. Obviously this disparity in dispositional options is greatest in cases involving intentional homicide, an offense typically punished by a sentence of life imprisonment or, in 37 states, death, and often carrying a mandatory minimum term far in excess of the dispositional period available to a juvenile court.

It is possible, of course, for discretionary decisions by prosecutors and courts to mitigate the severity of the penalty

195

for youthful offenders in criminal courts and thereby to close the gap between the dispositional consequences of delinquency adjudication and criminal conviction. Plea bargaining can reduce the level of the offense charged, and special sentencing provisions for youthful offenders may prescribe less severe penalties—and afford greater flexibility—than is available under the generally applicable sentencing provisions. However, because only a few states have enacted such youth offender statutes, sentencing leniency is dependent in most jurisdictions on the willingness of prosecutors and sentencing judges to regard the offender's youthfulness as a mitigating factor.

It has often been supposed that juveniles tried in criminal court are sentenced leniently as compared with older defendants, thereby bringing their sentences into line with the sanctions that would have been imposed in juvenile court. In order to test this so-called "leniency hypothesis," it is necessary 1) to compare sentences received by similarly situated juveniles retained and transferred by juvenile courts and 2) to compare sentences received in criminal courts by transferred juveniles with those received by older defendants convicted of similar offenses.

The available data do not, in fact, support the "leniency hypothesis." Rudman et al. (1986) studied 138 youths charged with violent offenses (murder, rape, aggravated assault, armed robbery, arson of occupied dwelling, and kidnapping) who were "considered for transfer" in the juvenile courts of Boston, Newark, and Phoenix between 1981 and 1984. (Unless the juvenile was charged with first degree murder, another criterion required for inclusion in the study sample was a prior "conviction" for a felonious offense against person or property.) About half of these cases were transferred, although the proportions varied significantly across jurisdictions. Conviction rates for the violent offenses charged were over 90 percent in both juvenile and criminal courts.

The data showed that the transferred juveniles were sentenced more severely than the retained juveniles in all three

196

jurisdictions. Of those transferred, 90 percent were incarcerated, as compared with 77 percent of the retained juveniles. Moreover, among the incarcerated offenders, the transferred youths received, on the average, sentences five times longer than the retained youths. Whereas only 17 percent of the retained youths received sentences longer than four years, 86 percent of the transferred youths received sentences in excess of four years. Not surprisingly, the largest differences in mean sentences were found in murder cases (247.5 months and 55.7 months for transferred and retained youths, respectively).

Although these data fail to support the leniency hypothesis, they do not conclusively disprove it. This is because of the problem of selection bias: Presumably the transferred juveniles represent those for whom available sanctions in juvenile court were regarded as insufficiently severe, and the retained juveniles represent those for whom the available sanctions in juvenile court were regarded as sufficiently severe. Thus, it is not possible to say, in the absence of a true experiment (randomly assigning juveniles to a transferred group and a retained group), that the two groups are actually comparable. Nor is it possible to say that the retained juveniles "would have" received the same sentences as those received by the transferred juveniles if they had also been transferred.

Surprisingly few studies have compared sentences received by transferred juveniles with those received by older offenders. In general, it appears that, after controlling for prior record known to the court, transferred juveniles (or young adults) are sentenced no more leniently than older offenders. Greenwood et al. (1984) studied sentencing patterns in criminal courts in Las Vegas, Los Angeles, and Seattle in cases involving offenders between 16 and 25 years old charged with armed robbery or residential burglary. They sought to determine how severely young offenders were sentenced in comparison with older offenders (and to determine how access to juvenile records of the younger offenders affected the disposition of their cases). In Los Angeles and Las Vegas, where adequate data were available to permit comparison, young adults (ages 18–20) were treated as severely as older offenders even when no effort was made to control for aggravating factors that might have affected their sentences. When offense severity (for example, use of a gun) and prior record were controlled for, young adults usually received *harsher* sentences (as measured by frequency of incarceration) than older offenders. (The only exception to this pattern was sentencing of burglars in Los Angeles.)

One study has focused on homicide. Eigen (1981) analyzed all cases involving juveniles arrested for homicides committed in Philadelphia in 1970. The study produced 154 juveniles arrested in connection with 63 homicides. The juvenile court retained jurisdiction in 79 cases (51 percent) and waived jurisdiction in the others. Of the juveniles retained in juvenile court, 61 percent were adjudicated delinquent, and only 49 percent of these adjudicated offenders were sentenced to institutions. Even among those retained offenders committed to juvenile institutions, the ceiling on confinement was the youth's 21st birthday.

Eigen's data demonstrate that the retained homicide offenders were sentenced relatively leniently by the juvenile courts. It is likely, however, that the decision to retain a case in juvenile court reflected a substantive judgment that "severe" punishment was not appropriate. Thus, for purposes of testing the leniency hypothesis, the key question is whether the transferred juveniles were treated with sufficient leniency to narrow the gap between the legally authorized punishments available to the juvenile and criminal courts. Eigen's data show, to the contrary, that sentence severity was about the same for transferred juveniles as it was for adults.

Among offenders convicted of killing in the course of a felony, 36 percent of the transferred juveniles were convicted of first degree murder (compared with 42 percent of the adults), subjecting them to a mandatory minimum sentence of life imprisonment, and all of the juveniles convicted of lesser degrees of homicide were incarcerated, with a median sentence length of three to five years. Among offenders convicted of a killing arising out of an altercation (rather than connected with a felony) few of the juveniles (7 percent) or adults (3 percent) were convicted of first degree murder, but more juveniles (58 percent) than adults (39 percent) were convicted of second degree murder. The higher rate of conviction for juveniles also translated into more severe sentences: more juveniles than adults were incarcerated (84 percent versus 73 percent) and more juveniles than adults received sentences in excess of two years (40 percent versus 23 percent). Probationary sentences were more likely for offenders with no prior record, but 19 of the 24 juveniles with no record received prison sentences, and one received a life sentence.

Eigen (1981) summarized his findings as follows:

> Almost 90 percent of the juveniles tried in adult court were sentenced to prison, but less than half of the juveniles tried in juvenile court were incarcerated. Three-quarters of the transferred juveniles would remain in prison when the last [retained] juvenile was released. Ten transferred juveniles were sentenced to life, one to death. (p. 1089)

Notwithstanding the possibility of discretionary leniency, then, the juvenile court's decision to retain or waive jurisdiction over adolescents charged with homicide has major dispositional consequences. In 37 jurisdictions a decision to keep the case in juvenile court precludes the death penalty, and in most jurisdictions it evades the mandatory sentences prescribed by law for anyone convicted of the highest grade of intentional homicide. Even if mandatory sentences are not prescribed, sentences received by most transferred youths convicted of intentional homicide are likely to exceed by many times the period of confinement available to the juvenile court —ranging from one year to six years, depending on statutory waiver age, juvenile court dispositional jurisdiction, and the particular offender's age.

Transfer Practice: The Determinants of Jurisdictional Choice

The stakes are high in the transfer decision, especially in cases involving charges of homicide and other violent offenses. Moreover, as was noted earlier, even young adolescents (14 or 15 years old) are eligible for transfer in most states if they are charged with murder. What, then, do we know about judicial practice? What proportion of the juveniles eligible for transfer are tried in criminal court? On what basis are these decisions made?

Arrests of Juveniles for Violent Offenses

We should first take a close look at the number of cases for which these questions are pertinent. Based on extrapolation from the arrest data filed by local police agencies with the FBI (U.S. Department of Justice 1985), about 1500 persons under 18 were arrested for murder or non-negligent manslaughter in 1983. (Eighty-eight percent of these youths were older than 14.) This figure represented about 8 percent of all arrests for murder and non-negligent manslaughter.

Although the focus here is on homicide, other offenses strongly implicating the retributive, deterrent, and incapacitative purposes of social control are rape, armed robbery, and aggravated assault. About 75,000 persons under 18 were arrested for these violent offenses in 1983. (Seventy-two percent of these youths were older than 14.) In contrast to homicide, however, juvenile arrests represented 17.2 percent of all arrests for these offenses.

Frequency of Transfer

Aggregated national data maintained by the National Center for Juvenile Justice (Snyder and Hutzler 1981; Kirsberg et al. 1986) indicate that between 5 and 6 percent of nondismissed cases in which juveniles are formally charged with violent offenses are transferred to criminal court, a proportion five times higher than for any other offense category. However, these figures are misleadingly low since the denominator includes *all* cases in which delinquency petitions had been filed, not only those in which the law permits transfer.

Findings from studies in particular jurisdictions focusing on small classes of transferable crimes suggest that the discretion to transfer is exercised in a significant proportion of cases and, not surprisingly, that transfer is most likely in homicide cases. For example, Keiter (1973) found that of the 174 homicide petitions filed in Cook County juvenile court in 1970, 44 (25 percent) were transferred. (In Illinois, the prosecution has the discretion to transfer, although the juvenile court has the rarely exercised authority to veto the prosecutor's decision.) In his study of juveniles arrested for homicide in Philadelphia in 1970, Eigen (1981) found that 49 percent were transferred. (It is important to note, however, that the class of persons charged with homicide in Eigen's study includes offenders alleged to be accomplices as well as the actual killers.) In a recent multijurisdiction study focused on a narrowly defined group of violent offenders "considered for transfer," Rudman et al. (1981) found that the juvenile courts of Phoenix, Newark, and Boston transferred 63, 31, and 20 percent, respectively.

The proportion of eligible cases waived in different states is undoubtedly affected by the basic variations in the juvenile transfer statutes. For example, the likelihood of transfer is clearly affected by the length of the juvenile court's dispositional jurisdiction. Snyder and Hutzler (1981) found that 16- and 17-year-olds charged with violent crimes who appeared before juvenile court judges whose jurisdiction terminated when the offender reached 18 or 19 were transferred about twice as often as similar offenders who appeared in courts whose dispositional jurisdiction extended until the offender was 21 or older. Similarly, after the Arizona Supreme Court invalidated a statute that had extended dispositional jurisdiction over adjudicated delinquents to the age of 21, transfers to criminal court tripled between 1979 and 1981 (Bortner 1986;

President's Commission on Law Enforcement and Administration of Justice 1967).

Snyder and Hutzler (1981) also found that courts with authority to transfer 14- or 15-year-old juveniles were more likely to transfer 16- or 17-year-old juveniles than courts whose jurisdiction over 14- or 15-year-old juveniles was exclusive. They interpreted this finding to indicate that "the 16- or 17-year-old offender may appear less amenable to juvenile court treatment to a judge who exercises that discretion in regard to younger offenders than to a judge whose amenability standard is derived from his experience with older offenders only."

Determinants of Outcome

On the face of the law, the juvenile court's decision whether to waive or retain jurisdiction requires an individualized predictive judgment regarding the likely behavioral effects of various dispositions available to the juvenile court. Even though the statutory criteria do not mention punishment, transfer decisions are undoubtedly influenced by punitive considerations; judges can hardly avoid asking whether society's interests in retribution, deterrence, or incapacitation can be adequately vindicated by the various dispositions available to the juvenile court (Keiter 1973). Indeed, some observers have suggested that community reaction is the major determinant of the transfer decision (Sargent and Gordon 1963). Thus, the articulated basis for the decision obscures the underlying tension between the competing paradigms.

Application of the statutory criteria is itself confounded by a latent tension between rehabilitative and incapacitative objectives. Although "public safety" or the offender's "dangerousness" is not everywhere mentioned as a relevant consideration in the governing statute, it is clearly taken into account by prosecutors and judges. Yet amenability and dangerousness do not always point in the same direction: an offender thought to pose a high risk of recidivism may also be regarded as a good candidate for juvenile court intervention, or at least not a hopeless one. Surely what every judge must ask is whether the juvenile court intervention is worth trying *in light of the risk and likely consequences of failure.*

Unfortunately, predictions about the likelihood of recidivism and the likely behavioral effects of alternative dispositions available to the juvenile court are little better than intuitive hunches, even when informed by clinical opinion. As Mulvey (1984, p. 195) has observed, "technical expertise" is "sorely lacking" and "little is really known about what will work with a given juvenile offender." Even the clinician's judgment is inevitably influenced by his or her beliefs about the relative desirability of a rehabilitative or punitive response. To the extent that judges rely too heavily on clinical recommendations, they are shifting to mental health professionals the responsibility for what is, and ought to be, a social and moral judgment.

These vague statutory criteria (for example, "amenability to treatment" in the juvenile system or "dangerousness") do very little to structure the exercise of judicial discretion. At the suggestion of the Supreme Court in *Kent v. United States* (1966) many states have prescribed a list of factors to be considered in making the transfer decision. Yet it seems generally agreed that these factors do very little to shape the ultimate decision, which must, in any case, be based on an individualized judgment. In a context in which the goals and values being pursued are so obscure, each judge must, in effect, legislate in each case. As Feld (1980) has pointed out, "Typical waiver statutes, couched in terms of 'amenability to treatment' or 'dangerousness,' are in effect broad, standardless grants of discretion."

From a normative standpoint, the prevailing system of individualized transfer decisions is functionally indistinguishable from the individualized sentencing system applauded by Justice Black in the quotation appearing at the outset of this chapter. It is, of course, subject to the same criticisms—inconsistency and arbitrariness—that have produced such widespread support for sentencing reforms aiming to reduce judicial discretion (Frankel 1973; von Hirsch 1976). It should not be surprising that some of the same disparities identified in criminal sentencing also have been documented in transfer decisions. Outcomes seem to be different for rural and urban areas within the same state (Feld 1980; Hamperian et al. 1982). Some studies have found that black offenders were transferred with greater frequency than white offenders (Keiter 1973; Hays and Solway 1972), although a recent study of transfer decisions in four urban jurisdictions by Fagan et al. (1987) found that the offender's race was not an independent predictor in three jurisdictions and had only a mild effect in the other. There is also evidence that offenders who kill white victims are transferred with greater frequency than those who kill blacks (Eigen 1981), a pattern also well documented in criminal sentencing, most extensively in capital cases (Gross and Mauro 1984).

I hasten to add that the empirical literature on transfer decisions is relatively sparse and is neither as extensive nor as sophisticated as the literature on sentencing (Panel on Sentencing Research 1983). Critics of the transfer process generally assume that findings about sentencing decisions are likely to be applicable to transfer decisions as well. I am inclined to make the same assumption. It should be noted, however, that there is some evidence that transfer decisions, in the aggregate, appear to be strongly influenced by a few objective factors such as certain aggravating characteristics of the offense (multiple offenses, possession of weapons) and the nature of the offenders' prior record (age of first offense, previous adjudication for violence, previous institutionalization) (Snyder and Hutzler 1981; Eigen 1981; Keiter 1973; Fagen et al. 1987; Osbun and Rode 1984). Of course, the same is true of discretionary sentencing. The problem there, which is likely to be true of transfer decisions as well, is that these factors do not account for a large portion of the outcome variance.

A few states have attempted to constrain transfer discretion through devices similar to those employed in the contemporary generation of sentencing statutes—by establishing presumptions favoring transfer in cases involving certain offenses or certain combinations of offense and prior record. The ultimate decision, however, remains individualized. Only one major investigation has been undertaken to assess the impact of this reform. In their study of the Minnesota legislation, which took effect in 1981, Osbun and Rode (1984) concluded that even though the frequency of transfer increased somewhat after the statutory change, the statute did not have a major effect on the selection process. They concluded that the statutory criteria were both underinclusive and overinclusive and that prosecutors and courts paid them little attention.

Summary

Let me now summarize the conclusions thus far reached before outlining some tentative views regarding reform of the transfer process.

1. The law governing disposition of juveniles charged with murder and other violent offenses has always reflected a profound ambivalence regarding the moral and social significance of the offender's youthfulness on the one hand and of the seriousness of his offense on the other. A contemporary shift in sentencing philosophy toward a just desserts paradigm, together with a pervasive concern about juvenile violence, has heightened this long-standing conflict.

2. Even though the juvenile court's jurisdiction normally encompasses offenders under 18 years of age, all states permit criminal court jurisdiction over 16- and 17-year-olds charged with serious crimes, and about three-fourths of the states permit criminal prosecution of 14- and 15-year-olds charged with murder.

3. Because of the wide variation in the dispositional authority available to the juvenile and criminal courts, and in dispositional practice as well, the choice of court is probably the most critical issue resolved in any case involving a murder charge.

4. In most states, where the choice of court rests on a judicial determination regarding the juvenile's "amenability" to

treatment (or "dangerousness"), judges inevitably take into account the retributive and deterrent purposes of punishment as well. Thus, the cases selected for transfer turn as much on the judges' values and intuitions as on any objectifiable criteria. To the extent that judges defer to the supposed clinical judgments of psychiatrists and other mental health professionals, the outcome turns largely on the clinician's own intuitions and values rather than any proven expertise.

Conclusion: Toward a Coherent Sentencing System for Juvenile Offenders

The law governing the jurisdictional borders between juvenile and criminal courts is unsatisfactory. It is impossible to justify the marked discontinuity between the dispositional consequences of juvenile and criminal court adjudication, a discontinuity that is especially pronounced in homicide cases. I am by no means the first to call attention to this problem (Twentieth Century Fund Task Force on Sentencing Policy Toward Young Offenders 1978; Feld 1978, 1980, 1983). Although space does not permit lengthy analysis of the issues that must be resolved in the effort to design a more satisfactory system, I do want to present an outline of my views on the shape of such a system.

1. The choice between delinquency adjudication in the juvenile court and criminal prosecution should be explicitly characterized as a decision about *grade* or severity of punishment, not as a choice between therapeutic and punitive intervention. As the President's Commission observed in 1967, juvenile justice is a system of social control, not a system of mental hygiene. Its separate existence is warranted not because of proven rehabilitative success but because leniency toward the young is morally justified and because the risk of failure is worth taking. As the Twentieth Century Fund Task Force observed (1978), "Protecting young offenders from the full force of the criminal law is prudent social policy." While vindicating the social interest in punishment, the law should provide

206

young offenders "with the opportunity to pass through this crime-prone stage of development with their life chances intact" (p. 7).

2. The transition from the lenient perspective of the juvenile court to the "full force of the criminal law" should be gradual. One birthday should not bring on the full force of the criminal law. Some categorization based on age is, of course, necessary. For example, there must be some point below which the moral basis for punitive intervention is so much in doubt that even delinquency adjudication should be precluded (Weithorn 1984; Weissman 1983). Where this line is drawn should turn on suppositions about moral development and evolving capacity for judgment and self-restraint. The Juvenile Justice Standards mark this point at the age of 10. There must also be some other point (age 21, for example) at which the offender's age ceases to carry any legal significance because it no longer carries any moral significance. But between these two points (say 10 and 21 years of age) severe and mandatory escalation of punishment based *solely* on the offender's age or *solely* on the offense charged should be avoided.

The major defect in existing law is that it reflects a major discontinuity in sentencing policy in the transition from juvenile to criminal court. As the Twentieth Century Fund Task Force observed in 1978:

> No single age during mid-adolescence should be used as a sharp dividing line for sentencing policies. [Policy makers must consider] sentencing policy toward young offenders in both juvenile and criminal courts and [must coordinate] the policies of these two institutions so that public policy toward young offenders is based on consistent and coherent premises. (p. 5)

3. The substantial gap in dispositional consequences now existing in many states should be narrowed. This can be done in either of two ways—by extending the dispositional jurisdiction of *juvenile* courts for some designated period beyond the adjudication (say three or four years) or by providing a distinct sentencing structure for "youthful offenders" in *criminal*

courts. The primary effects of "youthful offender" statutes should be to authorize placement in separate age-segregated facilities and to exempt the young offender from the imposition of mandatory sentences otherwise prescribed by the penal law. (An age-linked model of judicial jurisdiction over adolescents and young adults is depicted in Table 4.)

To the extent that the dispositional consequences of the jurisdictional choice are narrowed by these two devices, there should be correspondingly less concern about the dangers of discretionary decision making in the transfer process. An individualized process, therefore, may be acceptable if the jurisdictional choice matters less than it does now.

4. To the extent that significant escalation of punishment continues to depend on whether the offender is tried in juvenile or criminal court, the class of transferable cases should be significantly restricted and the jurisdictional choice should be governed by objective criteria relating to age, offense, and prior record, not by individualized predictive judgments. With one exception (to be mentioned below), clinical opinion should play no role in the transfer decision and should be confined instead to dispositional recommendations.

The seriousness of the offense should not ordinarily be sufficient, standing alone, to shift jurisdiction. However, in cases in which an older adolescent (16 or 17 years of age) charged with a violent crime also has a prior adjudication of serious criminal violence, the social interests in retribution and incapacitation may require more severe punishment than the juvenile system is authorized to impose (even if the juvenile court is given extended dispositional authority). The legislature would be justified in requiring transfer in such cases.

5. I can envision two major objections to this scheme, both of which call attention to the underlying ambivalence in our shared attitudes toward youth and punishment. First is the paradigmatic case of homicide. I have said that the seriousness of the offense, by itself, should not be sufficient grounds for transfer. But, it may be asked, what about the truly aggravated offense for which the sanctions available to the juvenile court

Table 4. Age-linked model of jurisdiction over children and young offenders

	Age	Jurisdiction
	21	Eligibility for sentencing under "young adult offender" statutes (exclusive criminal court jurisdiction)
	20	
	19	
	18	
Maximum age of juvenile court jurisdiction (18)	17	Overlapping juvenile and criminal court jurisdiction for serious offenses (zone of transfer)
Minimum age of criminal court jurisdiction (16)	16	
	15	Exclusive juvenile or family court jurisdiction (delinquency or *parens patriae*)
	14	
	13	
	12	
Minimum age of delinquency jurisdiction (11)	11	
	10	Exclusive juvenile or family court jurisdiction (*Parens patriae* only) (Neglect or ungovernability)
	9	
	8	
	7	

(even with extended dispositional authority) would be regarded as insufficient to express the retributive sentiments of the community?

Here is my response, together with a slight modification of my proposal. As long as significant dispositional consequences turn on the jurisdictional choice, it is unwise to *require* transfer of the entire class of murder cases involving offenders over a designated age. A generic exception for murder or intentional homicide is overinclusive because it would fail to take into account the clinically and morally significant variations among juvenile homicide offenders (Cornell et al. 1987; see also Chapters 2 and 3). Many, if not most, of these cases belong in the juvenile court because the interventions available to the juvenile court are adequate to effect the social purposes of punishment. As Cornell et al. have shown, offenders who commit "conflict" homicides are distinguishable in prior adjustment and history from those who commit homicides in the context of other criminal activity. In many of these situations, the punishments available to the juvenile court are sufficiently severe to serve the retributive aims of the penal law and the risk of recidivism is so remote that the incapacitating functions of penal intervention are not implicated.

So why not permit the juvenile court to make individualized judgments regarding the suitability of juvenile court intervention (in terms of the social purposes of punishment) in light of the circumstances of the offense and the offenders' prior adjustment and history? Unfortunately, if transfer in homicide cases were discretionary, this plan would reintroduce the dangers of arbitrary decisions that plague the system as it is. This is unacceptable. Here is my concession, however. If the legislature defines, in advance, specific characteristics of aggravated murder that reasonably justify more severe punishment than is available to the juvenile court, then waiver should be permitted based on offense alone. Most legislatures already have at hand a narrowed classification of aggravated homicide in their capital sentencing statutes. The retributive and deterrent judgments reflected in these statutes would seem to apply in the present context because they identify those aspects of homicide (for example, contemporaneous felony, torture, multiple killings) that are thought to justify an increase in the generally available punishment.

The second problem with my proposal is that I have said that transfer should be mandatory in cases involving a juvenile charged with a violent offense who has previously been "convicted" of such an offense. Here the objection will be that this classification could be overinclusive and that discretionary exceptions should be permitted to take account of the unique circumstances of particular cases—that is, cases in which the social purposes of punishment would be adequately served by the sanctions available to the juvenile court notwithstanding occurrence of the previous offense. I am prepared to allow the scheme to be presumptive, as long as transfer hearings are mandatory and judges are required to justify, on the record, decisions to retain jurisdiction. Under such a presumptive scheme, clinical opinion regarding the juvenile's development, maturity, and future prospects would be admissible.

6. Finally, a few words about the death penalty. On September 11, 1985, Texas executed Charles Rumbaugh, who had robbed and killed a jeweler when he was 17. On January 10, 1986, South Carolina executed James Terry Roach for his role in a brutal rape-murder of a teenager and her companion; Roach had also been 17 when he committed the crime. Rumbaugh and Roach were the first persons to be executed in this country since 1964 for crimes committed while juveniles.

Only 10 of the 37 states with capital punishment categorically preclude execution of offenders who were under 18 at the time of their crimes (Streib 1986). Of the more than 2000 prisoners on death row in May 1988, about 40 had committed their offenses while juveniles (Lewis et al. 1986).

The Supreme Court has been urged to rule that execution of offenders who committed their offenses while juveniles (that is, while under the age of 18) is unconstitutionally excessive. A majority of the Court appears to have concluded in *Thompson v. Oklahoma*, decided in June of 1988, that execution of a person for an offense committed while under 16 is unconstitutional. Four justices reached this conclusion. The fifth vote was provided by Justice O'Connor, who took the position that execution of a 15-year-old was unconstitutional in the absence of an explicit legislative judgment that offenders younger than 16 should be subject to the death penalty. Although she left open the possibility, such explicit legislative authorization in more than a few states would seem unlikely.

A judicial ban on executing older juveniles is unlikely to win the support of five justices. I suspect that the view expressed by Justice Scalia, in his dissenting opinion in *Thompson*, will eventually prevail in a case involving a juvenile who was 16 or 17 at the time of the offense.

In Justice Scalia's view, "There is no rational basis for discerning in [the rarity of juvenile executions] a societal judgment that no one so much as a day under 16 can *ever* be mature and morally responsible enough to deserve [the death] penalty. . . . " Even Justice O'Connor, who joined the majority in *Thompson*, was unwilling to endorse the proposition that juveniles under the age of 16, as a class, "are incapable of the moral culpability that would justify the imposition of capital punishment." All that can be said with moral confidence is that most adolescents are less responsible than many adults. But some older adolescents are more responsible than many adults, and some adults are less responsible than others. The problem, of course, is that the offender's age is only an indicator, not a test or measure, of responsibility.

The constitutional objection to execution of juveniles could be formulated, more generally, as a claim that the death penalty is a constitutionally excessive punishment for any defendants, regardless of age, whose capacity to appreciate the wrongfulness of their conduct or to conform their conduct to the requirements of the law was significantly impaired due to developmental immaturity. Although this approach might be pressed in subsequent litigation, the Court is unlikely to endorse the admittedly arbitrary proposition that 18-year-old juveniles may be executed even though 17-year-olds are constitutionally exempt.

To say that the line between 17 and 18 years of age has no constitutional significance is not to say that legislators should not draw such a line. Eighteen is a morally defensible line for the same reason that it offers a defensible jurisdictional boundary for the juvenile court's delinquency jurisdiction. Drawing imperfect but defensible lines is what the legislative process is about.

It appears, however, that many legislators have not been persuaded by a "this line is more defensible than any other line" argument. The common legislative judgment appears to be that some 17-year-old (or 16- or 15-year-old) killers are even more deserving of the death penalty than older offenders and the law should permit execution in such cases if the jury is persuaded that the offender's youthfulness carries little mitigating weight.

It is hard to argue with this judgment on its own terms. But I want to offer a different argument against the execution of juveniles, one that proceeds not from premises about the moral legitimacy and social value of the death penalty but rather from the premises about continuity in sentencing outlined in this chapter. The central problem with the death penalty for juveniles is that it exaggerates the disparity between the sentences available in juvenile and criminal court, and thereby distorts the process of jurisdictional choice in all cases for which the death penalty is potentially available. To promote the graded approach to juvenile sentencing outlined above, the death penalty must be unavailable in any case initially within the jurisdiction of the juvenile court.

This argument would not apply, of course, if the legislature were to make criminal court jurisdiction exclusive in cases in which juveniles older than a designated age have been charged with murder or with one of the aggravated types of murder punishable by death. It is revealing, however, that most states have not done this. They have, in effect, allowed the juvenile court to exercise a preemptive veto over the death penalty. Opponents of the death penalty would undoubtedly prefer a system that permits this discretionary juvenile court veto to one in which criminal court jurisdiction is mandatory in all capital cases. However, this discontinuity is too much for the system, or for juvenile judges, to bear. Whether juveniles otherwise within the jurisdiction of the juvenile court should be punishable by death is a judgment legislators should make one way or the other. On this issue, at least, the ambivalence should not be left unresolved. Even the American Bar Association, which has refused to take a position on the death penalty, has urged legislatures to preclude the death penalty for offenders under 18 (American Bar Association 1986). So do I.

References

Allen F: The Borderland of Criminal Justice. Chicago, IL, University of Chicago Press, 1964

American Bar Association: Resolution adopted by the house delegates, August 1986

Barrows S: Children's Courts in the United States, 1904. Reprinted in Foundations of Criminal Justice Series. New York, AMS Press, 1973

Bortner M: Traditional rhetoric, organizational realities: remand of juveniles to adult court. Crime and Delinquency 32:53–73, 1986

Cal. Penal Code, Annot. Cal. Codes Sec. 1170(a)(1) (West 1985)

Cornell D, Benedek D, Benedek E: Juvenile homicide: prior adjustment and a proposed typology. Am J Orthopsychiatry 57:383–393, 1987

Eigen J: Punishing youth homicide offenders in Philadelphia. Journal of Criminal Law and Criminology 72:1072–1093, 1981

Fagan J, Forst M, Vivon TS: Racial determinants of the judicial transfer decision: prosecuting violent youth in criminal court. Crime and Delinquency 33:259–286, 1987

Feld B: Reference of juvenile offenders for adult prosecution: the legislative alternative to asking unanswerable questions. Minnesota Law Review 62:515–618, 1978

Feld B: Juvenile court legislative reform and the serious young offender: dismantling the rehabilitative ideal. Minnesota Law Review 65:167–242, 1980

Feld B: Delinquent careers and criminal policy. Criminology 21:195–212, 1983

Frankel M: Criminal Sentences: Law Without Order. New York, Hill and Wong, 1973

Greenwood F, Abrahamse A, Zimring F: Factors affecting sentence severity for young adult offenders. Santa Monica, CA, Rand Corp, 1984

Gross S, Mauro B: Patterns of death: an analysis of racial disparities in capital sentencing and homicide victimization. Stanford Law Review 37:25–153, 1984

Hamperian D, Estep L, Muntean S, et al: Major Issues in Juvenile Justice Information and Training: Youth in Adult Courts: Between Two Worlds. Columbus, OH, Academy for Contemporary Problems, 1982

Hays J, Solway K: The role of psychological evaluation in certification of juveniles for trial as adults. Houston Law Review 9:709–715, 1972

In re Davis, 17 Md App. 98, 299 A.2d 856, 1973

Keiter R: Criminal or delinquent? A study of juvenile cases transferred to the criminal court. Crime and Delinquency 19:528–538, 1973

Kent v. United States, 383 U.S. 541, 546, 1966

Krisberg B, Schortz I, Litsby P, et al: The watershed of juvenile justice reform. Crime and Delinquency 32:5–38, 1986

Lewis D, Pincus J, Bard B, et al: Neuropsychiatric, psychoeducational, and family characteristics of 14 juveniles condemned to death in the United States, in Brief of the American Society for Adolescent Psychiatry and the American Orthopsychiatric Association as *amici curiae* in *Thompson v. Oklahoma*, No. 86–6169, S.C. May 15, 1986

Mack J: The juvenile court. Harvard Law Review 23:104–122, 1909

McKenna J, Grossman P Jr: Problems of modern juvenile delinquency legislation. Marquette Law Review 26:175–186, 1942

Mulvey E: Judging amenability to treatment in juvenile offenders: theory and practice, in Children, Mental Health and the Law. Edited by Reppucci ND, Weithorn L, Mulvey E, et al. Beverly Hills, CA, Sage Publications, 1984

O'Connel J: Jurisdiction—juvenile court v. criminal court. Journal of Criminal Law and Criminology 27:448–451, 1937

Osbun L, Rose P: Prosecuting juveniles as adults. Criminology 22:187–202, 1984

Panel on Sentencing Research, Committee on Research on Law Enforcement and the Administration of Justice, Commission on Behavioral and Social Sciences and Education, National Research Council: Research on Sentencing: The Search for Reform. Edited by Blumstein A, Cohen J, Martin S, et al. Washington, DC, National Academy Press, 1983

President's Commission on Law Enforcement and Administration of Justice: Task Force Report: Juvenile Delinquency and Youth Crime. Washington, DC, U.S. Government Printing Office, 1967

Rudman C, Hartstone E, Fagan J, et al: Violent youth in adult court: process and punishment. Crime and Delinquency 32:75–96, 1986

Sargent D, Gordon D: Waiver of jurisdiction. Crime and Delinquency 9:121–128, 1963

Snyder H, Hutzler J: The Serious Juvenile Offender: The Scope of the Problem and the Response of Juvenile Courts. Pittsburgh, PA, National Center for Juvenile Justice, 1981

Streib V: The eighth amendment and capital punishment of juveniles. Cleveland State Law Review 34:363–399, 1986

Twentieth Century Fund Task Force on Sentencing Policy Toward Young Offenders: Report of the Task Force, in Confronting Youth Crime. New York, Holmes and Meier Publishers, 1978

U.S. Department of Justice, Federal Bureau of Investigation: Crime in the U.S. 1983, in Sourcebook of Criminal Justice Statistics. Edited by McGarrel E, Flanagan T. Washington, DC, U.S. Government Printing Office, 1985

von Hirsch A: Doing Justice. New York, Hill and Wong, 1976

Weissman J: Toward an integrated theory of delinquency responsibility. Denver Law Journal 60:485–518, 1983

Weithorn L: Children's capacities in legal contexts, in Children, Mental Health, and the Law. Edited by Reppucci ND, Weithorn L, Mulvey E, et al. Beverly Hills, CA, Sage Publications, 1984

Williams v. New York, 338 U.S. 241, 248–249, 1949

Wolfgang M, Riglio R, Sellin T: Delinquency in a Birth Cohort. Chicago, IL, University of Chicago Press, 1972

Chapter 9

Treatment of the Homicidal Adolescent

ELISSA P. BENEDEK, M.D.
DEWEY G. CORNELL, Ph.D.
LOIS STARESINA, A.M.L.S.

Treatment of the Homicidal Adolescent

*T*he psychiatric treatment of the adolescent who commits homicide has not received adequate attention in the mental health literature. The literature in regard to treatment planning and treatment suffers from the same deficiencies as does the general literature in regard to adolescent homicide. Broad therapeutic principles are lacking or absent. In addition, much of the debate in the literature has focused on the initial referral from the criminal justice system, with primary concern being the appropriateness of either punishment or treatment (Benedek 1985). In this chapter, we address treatment planning in a more structured and organized fashion. We also address differential treatment planning by mental health professionals for three groups: 1) mentally ill offenders, 2) youngsters who commit homicide related to family or peer conflict, and 3) youngsters who commit homicide during the commission of another crime (Cornell et al. 1987a, 1987b; see also Chapter 3).

Diagnostic Evaluation and Treatment Planning

Before planning a course of treatment, it is critical that an adequate diagnostic evaluation be conducted. Unfortunately, many adolescents are not referred for a complete or adequate diagnostic evaluation. Factors such as social class, availability of resources, community reaction, heinousness of the crime, and legal strategy enter into the decision to request a psychiatric/psychological or medical examination. For example, during the course of our work, it appeared that a higher proportion of offenders from suburban or rural areas were referred for evaluation at the Michigan Center for Forensic Psychiatry. In suburban and rural areas, adolescent homicide was a rare event. In those areas it seemed as though court personnel believed that a homicidal youngster must be seriously disturbed. Thus, this belief generally resulted in a request for psychiatric/ psychological evaluation. In contrast, murder in Detroit's Wayne County is not a rare event (*Kids kill, kids die* 1986). Urban county youngsters were not necessarily referred for psychiatric evaluation, particularly if they had a long juvenile court record and the offense was considered only part of a series of crimes.

A complete clinical evaluation is critical for a beginning understanding of the underlying dynamics, motivation, and etiology of adolescent homicide. The diagnostic evaluation provides the essential clinical data that allow the clinician to decide whether psychiatric/psychological treatment is essential, appropriate, or potentially beneficial. For example, for the grossly psychotic or depressed youngster who kills in the midst of a psychiatric crisis, it would seem that psychiatric treatment is essential prior to his or her active participation in the criminal justice system. In contrast, the antisocial youngster with a long history of violent behavior is not a good candidate for intensive psychiatric treatment.

For another group of youngsters, a brief period of intensive treatment focusing on symptoms associated with guilt and shame might be helpful. Still another group might require only a brief educational intervention in an attempt to broaden their understanding of court procedures. An evaluation also allows the clinician to determine a possible location (jail, outpatient clinic, hospital) for treatment and to consider a variety of treatment modalities. In addition, it affords the clinician an opportunity to consider other diagnostic evaluations, including laboratory tests and sophisticated radiological evaluations.

Janowski and Mutter (1986) summarized the following essentials in any diagnostic evaluation, which can be applied to the specific case of adolescent homicide.

1. Chief complaint (homicide).   Here, the clinician should obtain a detailed history of the circumstances of the alleged homicide. For example, was the homicide planned or impulsive, was it secondary to another criminal activity or primary, was it symptomatic of a mental illness/emotional disorder or sociopathy? The patient/defendant's version of the act, his/her thoughts, feelings, and ideas at the time of the act should be elicited. Ingestion of drugs, alcohol, and controlled substances are also relevant.

2. History of present illness.   This includes important variables prior to the actual commission of the homicidal act. It is critical to assess the specific social circumstances of a particular homicide. Has the youth been involved in other conflicts with the victim? What is the history of their relationship? In a broader context, it is important to know the youth's current family and living situation, and the status of his/her most important relationships (with family, peers, and others) at the time of the homicide. It is useful to determine any recent stressful life events or circumstances that may have had a direct or indirect precipitating role in the offense. A surprising number of youths appear to have experienced recent disappointments in dating relationships or failures in school prior to their homicidal behavior. Often, the youth's seemingly inexplicable hostility toward the victim takes on added significance in the context of other relationships or stresses in the adolescent's life at the time.

   The history of present illness also would include a more general history of prior violent behavior. What has provoked past episodes of violence, for example, threats or insults, humiliation, anger, frustration? How chronic has the violent behavior been in the past? Is it limited to one instance, or is there a long history of violent behavior? Here, other signs and symptoms of mental illness or emotional disorder also are important. Has violence been associated with specific symptoms or signs of mental illness? With alcohol or drug intoxication? In addition, a detailed evaluation of family circumstances and past criminal behavior may help to sort out and clarify the youth's history of violent behavior.

Elucidating the circumstances and specific recipients (for example, peers, parents, authorities, the elderly) of past violence is critical for treatment planning. This information, along with detailed descriptions of the circumstances and emotions leading to past violence, will provide critical data for the treatment milieu and staff.

3. Past history. This includes a review of biological, psychosocial, and cognitive development prior to the homicide. Family history includes psychosocial history, genetic history, and a detailed exploration of relationships with parents and siblings. Here, special attention must be paid to family criminal history, medical history, and prior psychiatric illness. In an adolescent, factors such as school history, work history, and peer relationships also are relevant.

4. Ancillary history. Additional data are collected from other people who have had contact with the youngster. Such people might include past mental health clinicians, school teachers, physicians, police officers, friends, and family acquaintances. Any relevant information from past medical and psychiatric records aids in putting together the pieces of a clinical jigsaw puzzle.

5. Clinical interviews with the youth. Several interviews with an adolescent who commits homicide generally are necessary. In our experience, a homicidal youngster may present a clinical picture that makes it difficult to establish trust and rapport at the time of the initial interview. It is important to bear in mind that frequently these youngsters have been questioned extensively by police, their attorney, or other authorities. These experiences may leave them too exhausted, troubled, or wary to engage in still another round of questioning.

It is essential for the clinician to clarify the purpose and nature of his/her contact with the youth, the limits of confidentiality, and the possibility of court testimony. This is absolutely essential for legal and ethical purposes, but also helps delineate the boundaries of the relationship and distinguishes the mental health clinician from others who have interviewed the youth.

Some youngsters present with a defiant bravado and insist that they wish to be punished in a prison setting. Others are clinically depressed and almost mute. Still others are terrified by their first contact with the mental health and criminal justice system. It is very difficult to obtain necessary and relevant data from an adolescent at the time of the first clinical interview. If a clinician is experienced and skilled, it is sometimes possible to begin to establish a minimally trusting relationship. In our experience, it is only after several interviews that youngsters begin to talk about the events of an alleged crime in detail and depth and with some degree of honesty. Finally, if a youngster's account of a crime differs from that reported by friends, relatives, or police agencies, it is only after several interviews that a clinician can confront an adolescent with differing versions of the same event.

6. Parent Interviews. Parent interviews provide an opportunity to compare the adolescent's own history of previous functioning with the parents' reports as well as permit an initial opportunity to assess the parents' ability to provide support and care for the child during the difficult trial process and subsequent treatment. Finally, an assessment of the parents' own state of psychological health or illness is informative. A recommendation for treatment of siblings or parents might follow.

7. Other Interviews. When possible, interviews with peers, especially girlfriends of male youths or boyfriends of female youths, can be useful. Peers often have a more detailed and revealing account of the youth's behavior prior to the offense than parents. The youth may have been uncommunicative and withdrawn at home but more open with friends and willing to confide his/her troubles. The clinician should gain permission from the minor and parents before conducting such interviews. It is natural for clinicians to be concerned about the effects of interviewing on other youngsters who know the defendant or even the victim, but in our experience, these interviews have not seemed to be unduly stressful and can be accomplished in a supportive manner. Frequently, these youths already have been interviewed one or more times by police.

8. Psychological testing. Testing can provide additional insight into the current personality and cognitive functioning of adolescent defendants. The youth's intellectual capabilities, judgment, and general level of maturity can be examined in a systematic, objective manner. Such information can bear on a variety of forensic issues, including competency to stand trial and juvenile status. In addition, testing can be particularly useful when the youngster is uncommunicative or when there are equivocal indications of significant psychopathology which need verification. However, special efforts to establish rapport are necessary before presenting the youth with a potentially anxiety-provoking array of tests. Many frightened juvenile defendants already feel insecure and under tremendous scrutiny; testing can seem especially intimidating unless presented in a nonthreatening manner.

Intellectual capabilities are best assessed by an individually administered intelligence test such as the Wechsler Intelligence Scale for Children (Revised), appropriate for ages 6 to 16, or the Wechsler Adult Intelligence Scale (Revised). Paper and pencil IQ tests suitable for group administration are not appropriate; they are generally less informative and less reliable instruments that measure a limited range of intellectual abilities. Educational or achievement testing is usually not relevant; if needed, school records usually suffice.

The Minnesota Multiphasic Personality Inventory (MMPI) is a useful, widely accepted personality questionnaire that is most often used with adults, but it can be administered to adolescents as well. The MMPI is particularly useful in forensic settings in determining differential diagnosis and in assessing the defendant's tendency either to exaggerate (malinger) or minimize psychopathology. A variety of adolescent norms are available (Archer 1987). Computer-generated scoring and interpretation services are commercially available, but users should be well qualified and familiar with the MMPI. The special circumstances of a forensic evaluation may render computer-generated interpretations less applicable because typically they are developed for use with a general mental health population. Because the MMPI is a lengthy questionnaire, some support and encouragement may be necessary to ensure that the youth persists in completing each item carefully.

The Rorschach is the most widely used projective personality test. It can be valuable in assessing the youth's potential for psychotic thinking and disturbances in reasoning, emotional maturity, and many personality characteristics. The psychologist is advised that inferences from the Rorschach (or projective tests in general) can come under strong criticism during court cross-examination if the test is used in a subjective or nonstandard manner. The Exner Comprehensive System (Exner 1986) offers a reliable, objective scoring system, as well as adolescent norms, which can provide a defensible basis for psychological interpretations.

Other personality assessment techniques can be helpful as adjuncts to clinical interviewing. The purpose of these techniques need not be primarily to obtain test scores but to assist in communicating with the youth. For example, sentence completion tasks sometimes offer a recalcitrant or inhibited adolescent an alternative way of expressing feelings and concerns. The youth's responses to selected items might provide a basis for initiating discussion on sensitive topics like family relationships or social anxieties. Similarly, story-telling tasks, such as the Thematic Apperception Test (TAT) or the newer Roberts Apperception Test for Children, not only can lend themselves to specific scores and personality interpretations, but also can help the clinician identify important themes and concerns to pursue later in the clinical evaluation.

9. The physical examination. A medical examination is often overlooked by mental health clinicians. Valuable clues as to underlying medical illnesses are available with a routine physical examination. Most youngsters who commit murder unfortunately do not see a physician, and the information available from standard blood, urine, and x-ray tests is not obtained. More sophisticated technology such as CAT scans and magnetic resonance imaging are rarely if ever used. Lewis repeatedly admonishes the criminal justice system and clinicians for overlooking organic and neurologic problems in homicidal youngsters (Lewis et al. 1981).

Treatment Options

After all these data are collected, a preliminary formulation that summarizes the youth's problems from a biopsychosocial perspective can be developed. Then a reasonable treatment plan can be considered.

Residential Therapy

After a decision for psychological treatment is made, the clinician must decide whether inpatient or outpatient treatment is appropriate. Generally, residential treatment in a structured inpatient setting provides the safest and most secure place for a youngster who is either emotionally disturbed or in the midst of a crisis following a homicidal episode. Although it is possible to treat such a youngster on an outpatient basis, it is exceedingly difficult. The youngster may become dangerous to self or others during the course of treatment as repressed memories emerge or as difficult material is discussed. The guilt and depression such a youngster experiences following a homicide makes him or her a prime candidate for suicidal ideation or suicide attempts. If the youngster expresses any active or passive thoughts of suicide, residential treatment is mandatory.

Although the initial treatment period may be brief, a diagnostic period in a residential setting contributes to an assessment of true suicidal risk versus malingering or manipulative behavior. It also serves to protect the adolescent. If medication is a consideration, hospitalization is also critical in the first phases of intervention. The structure of an inpatient unit, as well as its ability to establish firm control, diffuses the intensity of aggressive impulses and supports a youngster in a crisis situation. Hospitalization as an initial stage of treatment for such youngsters is suggested by Pfeffer (1980), Petti (1985), and Haizlip et al. (1984).

In recent years there has been considerable interest in a variety of treatment approaches for aggressive youths that are most commonly implemented in institutional settings (Keith 1984). Behavioral approaches include the use of token economies and behavioral contracting familiar to many institutions for delinquent youths, as well as the use of time-out procedures and other forms of mild punishment.

Navacco (1975) has applied principles of cognitive behavior therapy to the treatment of aggression. This approach is predicated on the assumption that aggressive behavior is mediated by the person's cognitive appraisal of, and angry reaction to, stressful situations or events. Patients are taught a variety of self-control techniques, commonly termed "stress inoculation training," that include cognitive restructuring of how events are interpreted, relaxation training to diminish feelings of anger, and social skills training to develop more adaptive means of solving problems and expressing feelings. There is empirical support for the use of behavioral and cognitive-behavioral approaches in dealing with aggressive youths in institutional settings, but their application in outpatient settings is far more difficult and limited by practical problems in implementation, monitoring, and control (Varley 1984).

Most inpatient treatment approaches for violent youths are aimed at limiting or controlling recurrent aggressive behavior that ranges from anger and verbal abusiveness to occasional assaults. Treatment of homicidally violent youths is complicated by the fact that the single episode of homicide is sufficient to merit concerted treatment efforts, yet many of these youths do not exhibit milder aggressive behavior often enough to be suitable for behavioral programs. Differences between chronically aggressive youths and those who commit highly infrequent, but extremely violent, acts must be recognized (Megargee et al. 1967) and may merit differential treatment approaches.

Finally, the youngster who commits a murder during the course of another crime is the least likely to need immediate hospitalization. Such a youngster is protected from community outrage in a secure setting such as jail or detention. In addition, once a youngster starts on the mental health route, it is difficult to convince well-meaning authorities that the appropriate interventions available to the mental health system have been exhausted and that, despite empathy or sympathy, scarce and valuable treatment resources must be conserved and used judiciously and appropriately.

Psychotherapy

Psychotherapy at the initial stages is primarily supportive rather than uncovering. In the psychotic youngster, the unconscious is close to consciousness, and contact with reality is so tenuous that it is critical to direct interventions toward strengthening defenses that are adaptive and discouraging defenses that are likely to exert a regressive pull. While dealing with the simple realities of a highly stressful and traumatic situation, the adolescent needs enormous support. That is to say, the criminal justice system with its complexities may be overwhelming, and a youngster may need support in negotiating the various bewildering procedures prior to trial and during trial.

Haizlip and colleagues (1984, p. 143) describe their experience in seeking advice about the advisability of treating an adolescent who committed homicide with uncovering psychotherapy. Prior to starting individual treatment with such an adolescent, they questioned supervisors and peers, "Would insight-oriented uncovering psychotherapy produce the reliving of the murder which might result with a second ego rupture?" and "Was the murder the result of a neurotic personality conflict in which he had acted out and which should be resolved in insight-oriented psychotherapy?" Haizlip's mentor advised him in the following manner, "Damned if I know what to do in that case, Tom. I've just treated the ones who have fantasized doing it, not the ones who have" (Haizlip et al. 1984, p. 143). Another consultation resulted in one of Haizlip's colleagues telling him about an experience with uncovering therapy in a patient who after the therapeutic contact "returned to his cell and mutilated himself with a razor blade." Haizlip reports his decision to "steer a supportive course" in treatment.

It is particularly tempting for the therapist to consider uncovering, psychodynamically oriented psychotherapy in a youngster who kills in the midst of family conflict. Here, both conscious and unconscious internalized conflict and psychodynamics often seem to be so apparent that helping the adolescent to understand dynamic conflict as the therapist understands it seems compelling. However, the generally good behavioral adjustment of these youngsters to the controlled residential setting belies the inner turmoil, guilt, anxiety, and depression that may torment these youngsters. The clinician can be misled by the adolescent's seemingly untroubled facade. The dynamics so readily apparent to a therapist may lead to more violence on the part of an adolescent whose control may be tenuous.

More extended and intensive psychotherapeutic treatment is usually best initiated after there has been resolution of the youth's legal situation. Otherwise, preoccupation with legal outcome and concerns about confidentiality impair the youth's ability to engage in treatment.

There are a number of psychoanalytically oriented case studies and reports of psychotherapy with juveniles who have committed homicide (Mack et al. 1973; McCarthy 1978; Miller and Looney 1974; Scherl and Mack 1966; Smith 1965; see also Chapter 1). A central feature of treatment becomes the youth's working through of the many aspects of his/her rage and disappointment in early object relationships (which became focused on the victim), gradually repairing a damaged sense of self, and strengthening the adaptive capacities of the ego. The concept of dehumanization (Miller and Looney 1974) may be useful in understanding the youth's ability to escape feelings of empathy, guilt, or other aggression-inhibitory mechanisms by selectively responding to targets of aggression as inhuman, unfeeling objects.

Biological Therapy

In addition to psychotherapy, the use of psychoactive medications must be considered in the treatment of the homicidal adolescent. The clinician must decide whether to use medication on a short- or long-term basis based on the previous diagnostic assessment and current clinical assessment. Depending on the diagnosis, one of a spectrum of psychoactive medications might be appropriate. Such medications would include anticonvulsants, neuroleptics, antidepressants, and minor tranquilizers.

Antidepressant medications. Antidepressants are the treatment of choice for the seriously depressed homicidal adolescent. The depression may be the effect of a long-standing depression or a situational reaction to the violence. In any case, a trial of antidepressants is appropriate, and therapeutic doses are indicated. The first effects of antidepressants are improved sleep, energy, and appetite and diminished anxiety. The youngster may become talkative and more cooperative in therapy. Observers, attendants, and forensic personnel may report increased interest in educational and ward activity and increased personal contact with staff and other patients. Subjective improvement in depressed mood may be slow, although ward personnel observe improvement in energy level, interest, sleep, and appetite (Tupin 1987).

Antianxiety medications. These medications are most useful for the anxious and agitated patient. They may be used short term when a patient is adjusting to an inpatient ward or to control the agitated patient. Antianxiety drugs may also be used for long-term control, because antianxiety agents are now considered useful adjuncts in the control of agitation associated with schizophrenia, schizoaffective disorder, or bipolar illness. Antianxiety medications have occasionally been reported to have a paradoxical effect and increase violence (Bond and Lader 1979).

Antipsychotic medications. Antipsychotics are generally used for schizophrenia and mania, but they may be used effectively for the short-term control of aggression, agitation, paranoid ideation, or nonspecific psychotic behavior. Care must be taken not to use them for long-term sedation and behavior control or simply to chemically sedate and restrain a youngster who is presenting management difficulties. The use of antipsychotics for the long-term management of schizophrenic patients is well accepted, but special care must be taken to avoid side effects. The long-term side effects reported in adults, such as changes in liver function, cardiac arrhythmias, and tardive dyskinesia, have all been reported in children and adolescents.

Antimanic medication. The most general use of lithium is for control of manic symptomatology and long-term prevention of recurrent bipolar illness (Sheard 1975; Youngerman and Canino 1978). Carbamazepine has been studied with adolescents (Post et al. 1984) and has also been considered effective in both the initial control of manic symptoms and the prophylaxis of bipolar symptoms. The use of these drugs in patients with personality disorders is not yet well understood, although they have been used occasionally with adults on an empirical basis. Carbamazepine in particular has been suggested for use in patients who have rage outbursts associated with hyperactivity or attention deficit disorder (Post et al. 1984).

A variety of miscellaneous medications including beta- and alpha-adrenergic blockers, anticonvulsants, calcium-channel blockers, and antiandrogen hormones have not yet been carefully studied or evaluated in adults or adolescents (Tupin 1987).

Medication is useful not only in treating the biological underpinning of an illness but also in facilitating the youth's response to ongoing psychotherapeutic interventions. Hospitalization allows more controlled and aggressive use of medication. It also provides an opportunity for careful monitoring of side effects and use of sophisticated laboratory facilities to titrate medication dose and medication response. In adolescents, as in children, it is critical to constantly assess not only the effect of the medication but also the possible side effects of medications, including but not limited to cardiac arrhythmias and sedation.

The short-term use of medication at the time of trial can be beneficial. In particular, antianxiety medication assists some youngsters through complex legal procedures. Although antianxiety medications have been found to aggravate violence in some patients and in some rare cases to produce paradoxical excitement (Bond and Lader 1979), the paradoxical effect of excitement has not been reported in adolescents. In general, long-term use of medication is most useful for the group of youngsters who are clearly mentally ill. The youths whose homicide occurs during family or peer conflict may benefit from short-term use of antianxiety agents. Careful consideration should be given to the use of medication in the crime group youths, and the potential for abuse and addiction should be considered.

Family Therapy

A special problem is presented by the families of children who kill. Sargent (1962, 1971), Petti and Davidman (1981), and Haizlip et al. (1984) describe adolescents who kill in response to a verbal or nonverbal parental command. These adolescents

234

act as the agent of the family in carrying out their homicidal wishes. Sargent suggests that understanding this dynamic and presenting it to the court may be used as evidence of extenuating circumstances in the child's behalf. On the other hand, once such a dynamic has been explicated, it would become difficult, if not impossible, to reintegrate the adolescent into the family if such is the ultimate desired outcome. Although the adolescent may be accepted back into the family on a superficial level, once he or she realizes and understands his or her role in the family (as the murderer), one would expect the adolescent to be furious at other family members. Petti (1985) describes supportive work with parents around the issues of having a homicidal adolescent. He notes the importance of supporting the family in dealing with community reaction and helping them with their own reaction to a death. He encourages the therapist to assist the parents in making necessary changes in their parenting skills and hints that such changes may be critical in preventing future homicides.

We also have observed families in which a hated family member has been killed by the adolescent acting out the wishes of other family members. In these families, the adolescent is often immediately accepted back into the family. Under the guise of empathy, tolerance, and support, family members work for a premature termination of treatment or discharge from the hospital.

Psychosocial Therapy

In the hospital, the adolescent is immersed in a therapeutic community that often provides a more appropriate repertoire of skills necessary for effective social functioning. Here, educational programs (both traditional and specialized), recreational therapy, and social skills training are available. Each of these therapies has been extensively described in the literature.

Of particular importance in many homicidal youngsters is being able to experience and tolerate intense emotions without acting on them. A variety of techniques ancillary to psychotherapy have been described, including helping youngsters to learn to feel and think, but then not to act. King (1975) emphasizes the need to teach impulsive homicidal youths to "read, to write, to comprehend basic skills." He suggests a "deliberate melding of learning therapy and process with mental health concepts."

Clinician Reactions to Juvenile Homicide

The juvenile murderer understandably stirs strong feelings in even the most experienced of clinicians. Review of his or her violent behavior may stimulate reactions of fear, horror, or anger or other deep feelings. Personal reactions to the juvenile murderer's often-traumatic childhood experiences may include feelings of sympathy, shock, or dismay. His or her defensive facade of denial, indifference, or simply oppositional resistance in face-to-face interviews may be confusing or just extremely frustrating. All of these reactions can compromise or bias clinical judgment. Psychotherapists are well advised to monitor their countertransference reactions to these youths. The use of supervision or consultation with colleagues is often desirable.

Arcaya (1987) has described three possible biases of clinicians who evaluate defendants for the criminal justice system: the helper bias, the prosecutorial bias, and the uncommitted bias. The helper bias is a derivative of the clinician's basic humanitarian philosophy and a stance that leads the clinician to side consistently with the client offender. He suggests this bias is based in, part on ambivalent attitudes toward authority among some mental health professionals.

Those clinicians who harbor a prosecutorial bias identify with the police investigator or prosecutor in their attitudes and skepticism toward defendants. They consider the defendant's behavior in a condemning rather than a clinical fashion. They assume a judgmental role and may see themselves as taking protective action for the good of the community when they emphasize the dangerous, venal, or criminal aspects of the defendants they evaluate.

The "uncommitted" clinician is incapable of independent judgment and unbiased professional opinion. These clinicians are uncommitted either to patient or community, instead responding to institutional and bureaucratic pressures. Their opinions take form only in compliance with the perceived expectations of their superiors in the mental health/criminal justice system bureaucracy.

Arcaya describes these biases as countertransference reactions, although this term may be used too broadly in this context (Cornell 1987). It is clear that the attitudes Arcaya describes exist in a variety of circumstances other than psychotherapy and may arise from a complex of social, institutional, and situational factors. Cornell (1987) has discussed the ethical implications of these biases for psychologists and has outlined areas in need of empirical research.

Countertransference. Any clinician working with homicidal adolescents must be particularly sensitive to issues of countertransference. We use the term countertransference here in the more restrictive sense to mean the therapist's form of transference in reaction to the patient, which can be detrimental to treatment. It also may be useful to speak of countertransference-like reactions that clinicians develop in the course of extended evaluations.

Inexperienced clinicians who have had little forensic background may overidentify with either the victim or the adolescent. Either path can lead to disastrous therapeutic results. If overidentification with the victim occurs, there may be an alliance with police and the adoption of a prosecutorial stance. The therapist and patient are at odds in this situation.

The inexperienced clinician may also become a crusader foisting his or her own views about punishment of young people on the court rather than treating a particular youngster. The therapist who overidentifies with the patient might concur with the anger and rage that the juvenile expresses at the "system" and never help him/her to accept responsibility for his/her actions. New clinicians also may be often overly empathic with the youngster who kills in the midst of a family crisis. That is to say, they might express their own outrage at a brutal or seductive parent.

Fear. Many clinicians are fearful of adolescents who kill. Some overreact and are unable to establish rapport with an adolescent who quickly can identify a clinician's fear that the adolescent may lose control. Violent youngsters, who are often themselves afraid of loss of control, are not reassured or supported by anxious clinicians and become more frightened. Other clinicians may respond by denying or repressing realistic fear. If the fear is legitimate and the adolescents are dangerous, the clinician unwittingly could place himself or herself in a life-threatening situation without adequate protection. However, if the youngster is not in danger of losing control, a terrified clinician can reinforce concerns common to many of these youngsters that they will lose control; thus, the clinician will not be helpful to such a youngster.

The therapist's preoccupation with personal reactions to the youth can prevent the adolescent from coming to grips with his or her own feelings and substituting a clinician's understanding for a personal understanding and resolution of feelings. If a therapist is too empathic and the juvenile is seen only as a victim, he or she may never assume responsibility for the act. In addition, he or she may never feel or confront guilt, anger, rage, and all the other negative affects he or she has experienced.

Directors of residential treatment centers for adolescents seem to be particularly vulnerable to countertransference feelings. In our experience, it is often difficult to effect an admission for an adolescent because mental health administrators of inpatient settings project their fears of recurrent homicide and voice concern that the adolescent might kill again and on "their ward." Although violence does occur in inpatient residential treatment settings for youths, murder of staff or a patient in a controlled inpatient setting has not been reported (Benedek and Criss 1980).

Voyeurism. Finally, in some situations, the details of the homicide are so bizarre and incomprehensible to a new clinician that therapeutic voyeurism—that is, a desire to review repeatedly details about sexual activity, bloody gore, injury, and mutilation—takes over and the clinician cannot regain therapeutic neutrality. More broadly, the therapist loses access to his or her total reaction to the patient in treatment, which can be a source of insight into the relationship.

Outcome

Very little is known about the long-term outcome of juveniles who commit homicide, but with few exceptions the limited follow-up information available is surprisingly positive (Cormier and Markus 1980; Duncan and Duncan 1971; Gardiner 1985; Medlicott 1955; Tanay 1976). Authors suggest that juvenile murderers tend to adjust well in prison, relate well to their families, and attain an adequate social adjustment after release from custody.

However, none of the available literature is sufficiently comprehensive to justify making these kinds of generalizations for the population of juvenile homicide offenders as a whole. It appears that many of the follow-up case reports of adolescent offenders who achieve these good adult adjustments are individuals whose crime was an isolated act of violence. These are youths who did *not* have a history of chronic delinquent or criminal behavior. More often, their homicides were motivated by interpersonal conflict with the victim, especially in the context of abuse or mistreatment by the victim. One could hypothesize that the outcomes for juveniles who commit crime-related homicides are much less favorable, and that the risk for future criminal and violent behavior is much higher.

One exception to the positive outcome literature is Foster's report (Foster 1964) of a highly controversial case of a 14-year-old who was convicted of murdering his two-year-old brother and then was sentenced to death. Found incompetent to stand trial, he was hospitalized for nine years. During this time New York Penal Law was amended to exclude prosecution of children under age 15. On appeal, conflicting psychiatric testimony variously described the young man as insane or malingering, but the testimony was inconsequential because the change in penal law was applied retroactively, and the conviction was overturned. Over the next eight years the subject accumulated multiple charges for larceny, assault, nonsupport of wife and children, and possession of narcotics. One wonders what his time in treatment/incarceration accomplished.

Hellsten and Katila (1965) reported a minimum of seven years follow-up information on four youths who committed homicide in Finland. None committed further violent crimes, although two had arrests for larceny. Unfortunately, no information was presented on the nature of any treatment rendered.

Corder et al. (1976) obtained follow-up information on 30 adolescents after a minimum of 2 years, and an average of 4.5 years, posthomicide. They reported particularly positive outcomes for adolescents who committed parricide as opposed to other forms of homicide. Those who committed parricide were reported to require minimal psychiatric intervention, and by the time of follow-up, 9 of 10 had been released from incarceration. Available information indicated that at least 8 maintained a good relationship with their families.

In contrast, 19 of 20 adolescents who murdered someone other than a parent remained incarcerated. Although statistical analyses are not presented, the authors report that the adolescents who committed parricide were generally less aggressive in prison than were the nonparricide adolescents. However, even the nonparricide adolescents reportedly adjusted well to prison, manifested a comparatively low incidence of aggressive behavior, and participated voluntarily in work-study programs.

These data would support our impressions that those who commit intrafamilial violence are often in the midst of a family crisis and are not at as great a risk for future violence as are other homicidal youth. Perhaps this risk would be increased if a similar combination of external circumstances and interpersonal dynamics reoccurs. For example, an acquaintance who is similar psychologically to a hated family member might provoke a previously homicidal adolescent who had access to a weapon.

Cormier and Markus (1980) followed up on 29 juveniles who were convicted of homicide and remanded to custody of either adult (15) or juvenile (14) corrections in the Greater Montreal area between 1950 and 1974. Most were reported to have had good outcomes, though details are not reported. Only 1 of these youths committed a second homicide, and 2 committed suicide (including the youth who committed a second homicide). The authors describe an additional four individuals apart from their sample who did commit a second homicide later in life and suggest that the second murders stemmed from unresolved emotional difficulties of adolescence that were reawakened in adulthood.

Interestingly, Cormier and Markus comment on the common observation that juveniles typically show little remorse or guilt after the murder. They hypothesize that adolescents block out their affective reaction to the homicide for defensive purposes because of the additional adolescent turmoil and immaturity that precipitated the homicidal act. They report that over a period of years the youths do acknowledge depression and guilt and slowly work through a mourning process. Leopold's autobiographic account of his years in prison following his conviction for murder at age 19 certainly supports this view (Leopold 1957). Leopold refused to write about the actual homicide, but he described his striking lack of remorse for the murder of 14-year-old Bobby Franks until years after the crime, when he finally developed feelings of depression and guilt over what happened.

Conclusion

In summary, treatment planning for adolescents who are mentally ill would include focus on residential treatment, neuroleptic medication, supportive psychotherapy, and long-term aftercare planning. Mentally ill murderers who are acquitted as not guilty by reason of insanity typically are committed for treatment under civil law. Initially, they may be treated in a highly structured, maximum-security setting. With significant and stable clinical improvement, they may be transferred to more routine inpatient settings. The emphasis should be on graduated decrease in the restrictiveness of the treatment setting, with careful observation and evaluation at each stage.

Eventual return of these youths to the community, even with adequate preparation for outpatient care, involves considerable deliberation. The assessment of their potential dangerousness to others is underscored by their offense. Understandably, legal authorities as well as hospital personnel may be very reluctant to permit hospital discharge, even with substantial clinical improvement. Although research (Monahan 1981) indicates a substantial tendency for clinicians to "overpredict" dangerousness among a more general forensic population, research specifically on homicidal youths is not available. Moreover, the most consistent predictor of future violence is past violent behavior.

The decision to relinquish close observation and treatment of a youth who has been homicidally violent merits thorough analysis and review. Primary among the clinical considerations would be: 1) the stability of the patient's remission from psychotic symptoms; 2) the patient's attitude toward treatment and willingness to continue any prescribed psychotropic medication; 3) the patient's history of violent or threatening behavior while in treatment, particularly as he/she has moved to less structured or less secure settings; and 4) the presence of daily, ongoing social support (responsible adult supervisors, semistructured or group home living conditions, opportunities for ongoing work or education, and so forth) available to the youth in an outpatient setting.

Treatment for youngsters who commit homicide in the midst of family or peer conflict would more likely focus on interpretive psychotherapy, residential treatment, and, eventually, careful discharge planning and family therapy. Factors similar to those considered in discharge planning for the mentally ill adolescent would apply here as well. Although the youth may not be on medication, his/her attitude toward treatment and insight into the seriousness of the problem are important.

Treatment for youngsters who commit homicide during the commission of another crime would focus on treatment designed to facilitate passage through the juvenile justice or adult court system, supportive psychotherapy, and brief treatment with antianxiety agents. The disposition and follow-up care of these youngsters might best be left to the criminal justice system, which has its own mental health treatment resources. The therapeutic techniques currently available do not seem to be helpful to juveniles whose primary problems are antisocial in nature, but therapeutic efforts within the penal system may be worthwhile.

From the foregoing material it seems apparent that the appropriate psychiatric/psychological treatment of the homicidal adolescent is a critical area that leaves much room for further research. Although we have postulated three subgroups of adolescent murderers, there is no available research that directly links specific treatment approaches to each subgroup. The existing literature and our own clinical experiences have allowed us only to speculate and hypothesize, but not to make definitive or truly prescriptive statements. Treatment planning for the violent juvenile is only in an experimental and investigative stage.

Attitudes Toward the Study of Violent Youths

Although society as a whole expresses concern about extremely violent youths, progress in research on etiology and treatment has been hampered by limited research funding in the area of mental health in general and by the diversion of available resources to other politically more compelling, but not necessarily more important, subjects. Because violent behavior is not a "disease" and poses many conceptual problems in definition, the need for organized, systematic research efforts is not easy to promote.

However, there are indications of increased awareness of and sensitivity to violent behavior as an important topic. One hopeful sign is the increased interest in child maltreatment and abuse. Mental health efforts aimed at prevention of child abuse and treatment of abused children not only call attention to the study of violence but also directly affect many of the youths who are at greatest risk for future violent behavior—as aggressors rather than victims. One other positive sign is the growing public awareness of victim issues and the importance of attending to victims' needs. Although present efforts are focused on treatment of the traumatized victim, eventually attention will extend to preventive issues and thereby to research on the etiology and prevention of violent behavior from its point of origin.

The public and the legal system share an ambivalent attitude about punishment versus rehabilitation of violent juveniles that also impairs research efforts. The current emphasis on punishment of juvenile offenders from a "just desserts" perspective may be associated with a devaluation of efforts to investigate and understand the etiology of violent behavior. Behavior that is viewed simply as "bad" is condemned and punished, rather than studied and examined from a scientific standpoint.

Yet perhaps the punitive goals pursued by the criminal justice system need not conflict with clinical research and treatment. The ultimate aims and goals of each are not necessarily mutually exclusive. Etiological research that leads to detection of youths at risk for violent behavior, and which is followed by validated preventive interventions, is still desirable from a social perspective that condemns and punishes violent youths. Even treatment efforts need not be incompatible with punishment, to the extent that prevention of recidivism still remains a desirable outcome from either perspective.

References

Arcaya JM: Role conflicts in coercive assessments: evaluation recommendations. Professional Psychology: Research and Practice 18:422–428, 1987

Archer RA: Using the MMPI with Adolescents. Hillsdale, NJ, Erlbaum Associates, 1987

Benedek EP: Waiver of juveniles to adult court, in Emerging Issues in Child Psychiatry and the Law. Edited by Schetky DH, Benedek EP. New York, Brunner/Mazel, 1985

Benedek EP, Criss MO: Violence in a forensic center. Unpublished study. Ann Arbor, MI, Center for Forensic Psychiatry, 1980

Bond A, Lader M: Benzodiazepines and aggression, in Psychopharmacology of Aggression. Edited by Sandler CA. New York, Raven Press, 1979

Corder BF, Ball BC, Haizlip TM, et al: Adolescent parricide: a comparison with other adolescent murder. Am J Psychiatry 133:957–961, 1976

Cormier B, Markus B: A longitudinal study of adolescent murderers. Bull Am Acad Psychiatry Law 8:240–260, 1980

Cornell D: Role conflict in forensic clinical psychology: reply to Arcaya. Professional Psychology: Research and Practice 18:429–432, 1987

Cornell D, Benedek E, Benedek D: Characteristics of adolescents charged with homicide: review of 72 cases. Behavioral Science and the Law 5:11–23, 1987a

Cornell D, Benedek E, Benedek D: Juvenile homicide: prior adjustment and a proposed typology. Am J Orthopsychiatry 57:383–393, 1987b

Duncan JW, Duncan GM: Murder in the family: a study of some homicidal adolescents. Am J Psychiatry 127:74–78, 1971

Exner JE Jr: The Rorschach: A Comprehensive System, 3rd edition. New York, Wiley Interscience, 1986

Foster HH: Closed files on juvenile homicides: a case report. Journal of Offender Therapy 8:56–60, 1964

Gardiner M: The Deadly Innocents: Portraits of Children Who Kill. New Haven, Yale University Press, 1985

Haizlip T, Corder BF, Ball BC: The adolescent murderer, in The Aggressive Adolescent. Edited by Keith CR. New York, The Free Press, 1984

Hellsten P, Katila O: Murder and other homicide by children under 15 in Finland. Psychiatr Q (Suppl) 39:54–74, 1965

Janowski J, Mutter A: Treatment planning, in Psychiatry. Edited by Michaels R, Cavenar J. New York, JB Lippincott, 1986

Kids kill, kids die. The Detroit News, December 30, 1986, p 1A

King CH: The ego and the integration of homicidal youth. Am J Orthopsychiatry 45:134–145, 1975

Leopold NF Jr: Life Plus 99 Years. Garden City, NY, Doubleday, 1957

Lewis DO, Shanok SS, Pincus JH: The neuropsychiatric status of violent male juvenile delinquents, in Vulnerabilities to Delinquency. Edited by Lewis DO. New York, S.P. Medical and Scientific Books, 1981

Mack J, Scherl D, Macht L: Children who kill their mothers, in The Child in His Family. Edited by Anthony EJ. New York, Wiley, 1973

Medlicott RW: Paranoia of the exalted type in a setting of *folie à deux*: a study of two adolescent homicides. Br J Med Psychol 28:205–223, 1955

Megargee EI, Cook PE, Mendelsohn GA: Development and validation of an MMPI scale of assaultiveness in overcontrolled individuals. J Abnorm Psychol 72:519–528, 1967

McCarthy J: Narcissism and the self in homicidal adolescents. Am J Psychoanal 38:19–29, 1978

Miller D, Looney J: The prediction of adolescent homicide: episodic dyscontrol and dehumanization. Am J Psychoanal 34:187–198, 1974

Monahan J: The Clinical Prediction of Violent Behavior. Rockville, MD, U.S. Department of Health and Human Services, 1981

Navacco RW: Anger Control: The Development and Evaluation of an Experimental Treatment. Lexington, MA, Lexington Books, 1975

Petti TA: The juvenile murderer, in Emerging Issues in Child Psychiatry and the Law. Edited by Schetky DH, Benedek EP. New York, Brunner/Mazel, 1985

Petti TA, Davidman L: Homicidal school-aged children: cognitive style and demographic features. Child Psychiatry Hum Dev 12:82–89, 1981

Pfeffer CR: Psychiatric hospital treatment of assaultive homicidal children. Am J Psychother 34:197–207, 1980

Post RM, Rubinow DR, Uhde TW: Biochemical mechanisms of action of carbamazepine in affective illness and epilepsy. Psychopharmacol Bull 20 (Summer):585–590, 1984

Sargent D: Children who kill—a family conspiracy? Social Work 7:35–42, 1962

Sargent D: The lethal situation: transmission of urge to kill from parent to child, in Dynamics of Violence. Edited by Fawcett J. Chicago, American Medical Association, 1971

Scherl DJ, Mack JE: A study of adolescent matricide. J Am Acad Child Psychiatry 5:559–593, 1966

Sheard MH: Lithium in the treatment of aggression. J Nerv Ment Dis 160:108–118, 1975

Smith S: The adolescent murderer: a psychodynamic interpretation. Arch Gen Psychiatry 13:310–319, 1965

Tanay E: Reactive parricide. J Forensic Sci 21:76–82, 1976

Tupin J: Psychopharmacology and aggression in clinical treatment of the violent person, in Clinical Treatment of the Violent Individual. Edited by Roth L. New York, Guilford Press, 1987

Varley WH: Behavior modification approaches to the aggressive adolescent, in The Aggressive Adolescent: Clinical Perspectives. Edited by Keith CR. New York, The Free Press, 1984

Youngerman J, Canino IA: Lithium carbonate use in children and adolescents. Arch Gen Psychiatry 35:216–224, 1978